Contentious Issues

of related interest

Social Awareness Skills for Children
Márianna Csóti
ISBN 1 84310 003 7

Incorporating Social Goals in the Classroom
A Guide for Teachers and Parents of Children with High-Functioning Autism and Asperger Syndrome
Rebecca A. Moyes
ISBN 1 85302 967 X

Helping Children to Build Self-Esteem
A Photocopiable Activities Book
Deborah Plummer
ISBN 1 85302 927 0

People Skills for Young Adults
Márianna Csóti
ISBN 1 85302 716 2

Group Work with Children and Adolescents
A Handbook
Edited by Kedar Nath Dwivedi
ISBN 1 85302 157 1

Listening to Young People in School, Youth Work and Counselling
Nick Luxmoore
ISBN 1 85302 909 2

How We Feel
An Insight into the Emotional World of Teenagers
Edited by Jacki Gordon and Gillian Grant
ISBN 1 85302 439 2

Contentious Issues
Discussion Stories for Young People

Márianna Csóti

Jessica Kingsley Publishers
London and Philadelphia

First published in Great Britain in 1995 by Whyld Publishing Co-op under the title 'Contentious Issues', in the form of three packs containing loose sheets for use in Personal, Social and Health Education.

    The material has been rewritten to form a photocopiable book suitable for a wider market with additional material and comprehensive Leader Sheets to enable any adult to run the discussion sessions. Please see p.12 for details of photocopiable material.

First published in the United Kingdom in 2002 by
Jessica Kingsley Publishers Ltd,
116 Pentonville Road, London
N1 9JB, England
and
325 Chestnut Street,
Philadelphia PA 19106, USA.

www.jkp.com

© Copyright 2002 Márianna Csóti

Library of Congress Cataloging in Publication Data
A CIP catalog record for this book is available from the Library of Congress

British Library Cataloguing in Publication Data
A CIP catalogue record for this book is available from the British Library

ISBN 1 84310 033 9

Printed and Bound in Great Britain by
Athenaeum Press, Gateshead, Tyne and Wear

Contents

Section 2

Section 3 195

Introduction 197

Summary of Contents 197

About the Book

Contentious Issues is a collection of short stories and exercises written to promote discussion and awareness among young people aged between eleven and eighteen, for use by professionals and parents or guardians. *Contentious Issues* challenges young people to consider events and the part they themselves play in life, encouraging deeper thinking and awareness of how their behaviour can negatively affect others, producing more responsible and independently thinking young adults.

The book allows moral viewpoints to be expressed in the security of discussion of a fictional event so that participants do not feel threatened or intimidated by being presented with a problem taken directly from their own lives.

The book is intended to foster:

- feelings of moral obligations
- understanding of positive social behaviour
- understanding of the consequences of negative social behaviour
- understanding that there are not always single 'right' answers
- awareness of how to approach problems in life and how to carefully consider the options open to oneself
- feelings of responsibility for one's actions and inactions
- awareness of where to go for help when one is out of one's depth
- acceptance that it is not a sign of failure to admit to needing help
- a true understanding of what maturity is, rather than a misguided belief that it is shown by unyielding, uncompromising behaviour
- understanding of human nature and how people feel about things that have happened to them
- awareness of the opinions of other people one is in session with
- an open mind that is prepared to listen to all points of view before finally being made up

- an open mind that is prepared to change opinions in the light of new information or understanding of what's involved
- a caring for oneself and for others.

Although the stories were written with group work in mind, it is possible to use these stories one-to-one.

The stories represent current comprehensive school life in a multi-ethnic environment and focus on the concerns of the children (aged 11 to 18). The stories are designed to challenge racism and sexism (and many other stereotyped assumptions). Although only three of the stories (stories 11, 27 and 33) deal specifically with race and gender issues, the characters come from a variety of cultural backgrounds. White and black children, for example, are equally in trouble, both displaying negative behaviour and suffering emotional difficulties, as are boys and girls.

This material enables students to think deeply about themselves and their attitudes and encourages them to modify any anti-social behaviour they may have. It also encourages those who need help to ask for it.

Sections 1–3 are concerned with a multitude of issues that affect young people generally, such as bullying (in its many and varied forms), criminal acts, addictions, health issues, questions of right and wrong.

Section 4 contains tasks as well as stories and has a single general theme – that of relationships, feelings and the inner person. Issues such as suicide, terminal illness, bereavement, marriage, teenage pregnancy, controlling relationships and decision-making are explored. These sessions are suitable for young people up to the age of 18. It is possible to use them for under 16-year-olds, if the material has direct relevance to the group.

Leaders' Notes

About one hour is needed to use each section of material productively. This, of course, can vary either way, depending on the ability and interests of the young people concerned.

The Leader should take a supervisory role, guiding participants back to the salient issues when side-tracked and making sure that time is spread over the whole of the material. However, if a special interest is sparked this can be returned to at the end of the session or on a subsequent occasion.

Time permitting, more in-depth thought may be provoked if the participants are in small groups – it is more likely that each will make a contribution in a smaller group and the quality of discussions may be better as their concentration may be more intense. However, if the whole group is small enough not to warrant sub-groups, time is saved by not needing to bring the findings together at the end.

Discussing emotive and contentious issues through stories takes the spotlight off those who may feel threatened by issues directly relating to themselves. Also, any decisions about appropriate and inappropriate behaviour are made not by someone in authority but by others in their own peer group, allowing participants to view a situation with objectivity and without the resentment of being dictated to.

The Leader is not expected to present the answers – possible solutions to problems should come from the participants themselves, developing their sense of the world and what is right and wrong. Also, to many of the questions posed there is not just one right answer. It depends on the circumstances and the personalities involved and the backgrounds of the individuals.

The Leader must be sensitive to the participants but not to the point of agreeing with everything they say. The suggested answers should be used by the Leader to challenge viewpoints (to allow the participants to reach a deeper understanding) or to spark off further discussion about the situation and offer tentative suggestions when the participants have run out of ideas.

A good working relationship between the Leader and the participants is essential.

Contact details have been provided for help or further information – either for the Leader or for the participants themselves.

The Leader Sheets are intended for Leader use only. Please note that any statistics or factual details refer to the UK only. If you are working in another country you may have to amend the answers suggested in the book (for example, the legal limit for driving under the influence of alcohol varies from country to country and in some is banned altogether). Also, the contact details given in the appendix are for UK readers only, although the websites can be accessed from all over the world.

Note

All Stories and Discussion Sheets are photocopiable by the person or persons within the institution that bought the book, as is the Appendix of Useful Contacts. The Leader Sheets are for Leader use only and may not be photocopied.

Section 1

Introduction

Section 1 is concerned with issues relevant to 11- to 14-year-olds. Stories 1–5 are interconnected with a developing theme and should be read in order, although each story is complete in itself. The rest of the stories in Section 1 can be read in any order. Some of the characters in the stories also appear in later sections.

Summary of contents

Story	Title	Subject
1	Joshua's Birthday Present*	Carrying a knife, 'grassing'
2	Not So Sweet Revenge*	Revenge
3	Goodbye Shaun*	Solvent abuse
4	Extortion!*	Extortion
5	'Atch Out!!*	Bereavement, disability
6	Science Test!	Cheating, pressure from parents
7	Hoi Ping Is Unhappy	Communication with parents
8	It Happened One Day	Phobias and panic attacks
9	Preeti's Lost Bracelet	Stealing
10	Just One Last Game	Computer games addiction
11	A Better Class of People	Racism
12	Slag!	Divorce/separation

*Titles in succession are interconnected and should be read in order.

STORY 1: *Joshua's Birthday Present*

Shaun, Hoi Ping and Rajesh were admiring Joshua's birthday present in the schoolyard before school. It was a penknife, but no ordinary one.

'Look,' Joshua told them, opening it out, 'it's a tin opener too. And it's got a corkscrew and a screwdriver end here,' he said, pointing to each special part in turn. 'This is one of the best you can get,' he informed them proudly. His father had told him that morning that it was a very good quality penknife and if he looked after it, it should last him for all his life. It was the best present he'd had.

Shaun looked at the knife with envy. Why wasn't he ever given something like that? He wished he'd got one.

Thinking about it in class, Shaun suddenly remembered it was against the school rules to bring a knife to school. That'll teach him, Shaun thought meanly, if it gets confiscated.

During registration after lunch, Mrs Price, their form teacher, called Joshua up to her desk. She quietly asked him about the penknife. Shaun busied himself with sorting out his books for the next lesson and pretended not to see.

Joshua went back to his bag to get the penknife to hand it over to Mrs Price. She told him she was going to phone his father. The whole class was watching him and he felt very embarrassed. His face felt as though it was on fire.

He'd only brought in his knife to show his friends. He now wished his dad had never given him the thing. He'd been told not to take it to school, but he thought that just this once it wouldn't matter. His dad would be furious.

On his way home he puzzled over how Mrs Price had got to know about the knife. No one had seen it apart from Shaun, Hoi Ping and Rajesh. And they wouldn't have told because they were friends!

The next day, Rajesh and Hoi Ping hurried over to Joshua as soon as he arrived. Joshua told them his dad had hit the roof because he'd had to go to school to pick up the knife. It had made him look like he was irresponsible giving such a present to his son and he was angry because it had made him look foolish.

Rajesh told him that he knew who had told Mrs Price. His sister, Sangita, had seen Shaun go into Mrs Price's room at lunchtime. So it had been Shaun who had told on him! Joshua couldn't believe it at first. Why had he done it?

Then Shaun arrived and, as he approached, his smile faded because they were all looking at him as though he had some kind of disease. He knew they'd found out. He'd wished he hadn't done it almost as soon as he'd come out of Mrs Price's room, but it was too late then.

'Why?' Joshua asked him.

'It was against the school rules,' Shaun replied. 'You shouldn't have brought it in.'

'He shouldn't have,' agreed Hoi Ping. 'But that's not really why you told was it?'

'He was jealous!' Rajesh exclaimed.

'I'm sorry,' Shaun told Joshua.

'I'm sorry too,' Joshua said. 'I'm sorry I brought it in. I know it was wrong but I didn't think it would matter, just the once. And I thought you were my friend. Friends don't tell.'

Discussion Sheet 1: Joshua's Birthday Present

1. (a) Why is it a school rule not to bring knives of any kind to school?

   (b) Is it a sensible rule?

2. How did Shaun feel after telling Mrs Price about the knife?

3. Have you ever done anything that you've later regretted?

4. Was it fair of the other pupils to ignore Shaun because he'd 'grassed'?

5. Was there a better way of letting Joshua know that he shouldn't have brought the knife to school?

6. There is an unwritten law that pupils shouldn't 'grass' on each other. Can you think of times when it is OK (or even advisable) to break that law?

7. How would you feel if your best friend 'grassed' on you? Would you try to understand why or would you stop being friends?

8. People make mistakes in relationships – right from childhood through to adulthood. Can your friendships survive misunderstandings or hurts, or do they break up at the first sign of trouble?

9. If someone wants to say sorry do you try to help out? Or do you make it hard for the person, to make him or her suffer?

10. What happens when your parents or guardians fall out? Do you copy their way of solving problems, or have you developed your own way of dealing with a hurtful friendship?

Leader Sheet 1: Joshua's Birthday Present

1. (a) **Why is it a school rule not to bring knives of any kind to school?**

    - To protect pupils from potential harm.
    - To protect staff and the general public. Even if the person bringing the knife to school does not intend any harm, it could be stolen from that person and then used by someone else.
    - To protect the school from possible vandalism.
    - Because it is an offence to carry sharp objects that can be used as weapons.

    (b) **Is it a sensible rule?**

    Yes, it is a sensible rule. It is for the good of everyone.

2. **How did Shaun feel after telling Mrs Price about the knife?**

    - Guilty.
    - Scared (of being found out).
    - Ashamed.
    - Self-hating.
    - He wished he could turn the clock back or undo what he had just done.

3. **Have you ever done anything that you've later regretted?**

    (Personal response required.)

4. **Was it fair of the other pupils to ignore Shaun because he'd 'grassed'?**

    Yes: People feel very strongly about being 'grassed' on. Human nature would make them want to punish Shaun – and as he grassed because of jealousy and not because he thought anyone was in danger, his friends thought he deserved their treatment. He had broken his peers' 'social rules' and so was being excluded.

    No: He should be given the opportunity to apologise and make amends rather than be ostracised.

5. **Was there a better way of letting Joshua know that he shouldn't have brought the knife to school?**

   Shaun could have reminded Joshua that it was against the school rules and it was too risky to bring it in again, and that someone might steal it from him.

6. **There is an unwritten law that pupils shouldn't 'grass' on each other. Can you think of times when it would be OK (or even advisable) to break that law?**

   - If the person was being a danger to himself or others.
   - If someone needed protection, for example because of threats, bullying or extortion.
   - If it was illegal in a big way. (Taking or supplying drugs.)

7. **How would you feel if your best friend 'grassed' on you? Would you try to understand why or would you stop being friends?**

   (Personal responses required.)

8. **People make mistakes in relationships – right from childhood through to adulthood. Can your friendships survive misunderstandings or hurts, or do they break up at the first sign of trouble?**

   (Personal response required.)

9. **If someone wants to say sorry do you try to help out? Or do you make it hard for the person to make him, or her suffer?**

   (Personal response required.)

10. **What happens when your parents or guardians fall out? Do you copy their way of solving problems, or have you developed your own way of dealing with a hurtful friendship?**

    (Personal responses required.)

STORY 2: Not So Sweet Revenge

'Start on a new page and copy the notes from the board,' Miss Atkinson told her science class.

Shaun rooted in his bag. 'Oh, no!' he exclaimed. He'd forgotten to bring his pencil case to school. It was the third time that week.

He had been in such a rush, barely having time to eat his cornflakes. He'd overslept again, having spent the night tossing and turning in agonies because he had told on his friend, Joshua, to their form teacher and Joshua had got into a great deal of trouble. And now they weren't talking.

'Have you got a spare pen?' Shaun asked Sally, who sat next to him. Sally shook her head.

'Ssh,' Miss Atkinson said.

Very quietly, Shaun tried to attract the attention of Joshua, who sat on a table next to his. 'Joshua,' Shaun whispered loudly. There was no response. 'Joshua!'

'Shaun, if you don't stop talking and get on with your work I'll keep you back at break.' Miss Atkinson's voice was stern.

'I haven't got a pen, Miss,' Shaun explained.

'Oh? Again?' Miss Atkinson was not impressed. 'Does anyone have a pen to lend Shaun?' she asked the class.

'Here,' Joshua got up and handed one to Shaun. He kicked Shaun's bag out into the aisle as he returned to his seat.

Shaun smiled with relief. He tried to write the date with it but nothing happened. Joshua sniggered. Shaun pressed the nib down harder but still had no success. 'It doesn't work,' Shaun whispered across to Joshua. 'Have you got another one?'

'Shaun, if you don't get on with your work soon, I'll write in your homework diary to your parents,' Miss Atkinson's voice boomed.

'It doesn't work, Miss,' Shaun told her sheepishly. The class giggled out loud.

'Let me see,' Miss Atkinson said, coming over to his table. She tripped on Shaun's bag. Joshua smiled behind his hand. He wanted Shaun to get into trouble just like *he* had the week before.

'Shaun Robinson, how many times have I told this class, and you in particular, to observe safety rules? Never, never, leave bags or coats for someone to trip up on. They should always be pushed under the tables or left at the back of the laboratory.'

'But it wasn't –'

'Shaun, I don't want to listen to any more of your excuses. You arrived late, you don't have the proper writing equipment with you yet again and you don't observe safety procedures. What if I had been carrying chemicals or hot liquid? There could have been a nasty accident! I'll arrange a detention at the end of the lesson. I've certainly given you enough warnings.' Angrily, Miss Atkinson gave Shaun her pen to write with, shoved his bag under the table with her foot and got the class to carry on.

Joshua gave Shaun a 'serves you right' look.

Shaun tried to concentrate on copying the work from the board, swallowing hard to stop his tears. The whole class knew he was a grass. They must hate him.

At lunchtime, Shaun sat miserably in the cloakroom quietly crying. Joshua found him and he realised he had been just as mean to Shaun as Shaun had been to him. But it was worse – he'd thought about how to get his own back and had done it deliberately to hurt Shaun. He'd come to say sorry but didn't know how to start.

'My dad had promised me a new bike if I went a whole year without getting into trouble. And now I won't have it, thanks to you!' Shaun shouted.

Joshua realised they weren't quits after all.

Discussion Sheet 2: Not So Sweet Revenge

1. (a) If you were to repay an unkind deed how would you go about it?

   (b) What does this achieve?

2. (a) Was what Joshua did fair?

   (b) Did Shaun deserve it?

3. Was Joshua as unkind to Shaun as Shaun was to him? Or was Shaun worse because he was mean first of all?

4. Would you have wanted revenge or would you have tried to patch things up?

5. Why do you think Shaun didn't tell Miss Atkinson at breaktime that Joshua had kicked his bag into the aisle?

6. (a) Did revenge make Joshua feel good about himself?

   (b) Have you ever done something similar? How did you feel?

7. Has someone ever taken revenge on you? How did it make you feel?

8. Was there a better way of Joshua getting his own back?

9. If Joshua wanted Shaun to stay his friend could he have shown how hurt he was in some other way?

10. Shaun blamed Joshua for him getting into trouble and not getting his bike for his birthday. Was this fair?

Leader Sheet 2: Not So Sweet Revenge

1. **(a) *If you were to repay an unkind deed how would you go about it?***

   - Not talk to the person.
   - Get the person into trouble.
   - Try to take the person's friends away.
   - Tell lies about the person.
   - Spread gossip about the person.

   (b) *What does this achieve?*

   - It would make matters worse between the two of you and it would be even harder to make up – as Joshua found.
   - You make an enemy.
   - There is bad feeling between the two of you.
   - Any pleasure you'd get from it would be short-lived.
   - Other people may not respect you as it is not a positive way to treat someone – and they wouldn't want to be treated like that themselves.
   - You lose a friend.
   - It could start a circle of revenge – you might have something done against you next.

2. **(a) *Was what Joshua did fair?***

   - It was unkind to get Shaun into trouble deliberately – and vindictive.
   - It was not fair because Joshua was not repaying like with like. The two situations were different – Joshua had done wrong, by both the school and his father, in taking the knife to school whereas Shaun got into trouble because Joshua created a situation of Shaun being in the wrong, by shoving out the bag that tripped up Miss Atkinson and giving him a pen that didn't write.

(b) Did Shaun deserve it?

(Personal response required.)

3. **Was Joshua as unkind to Shaun as Shaun was to him? Or was Shaun worse because he was mean first of all?**

Shaun did start the problems in their friendship, but Joshua has nothing to be proud of either. They both did wrong and should now concentrate on becoming friends again. Being judgemental isn't positive behaviour. One could argue that either one was worse. (Shaun for starting it, Joshua for deliberately getting Shaun into trouble with Miss Atkinson more than once.)

4. **Would you have wanted revenge or would you have tried to patch things up?**

(Personal response required.) (Revenge can only make things worse and if you care about someone it is better to try and get back to a pleasant footing as soon as possible.)

5. **Why do you think Shaun didn't tell Miss Atkinson at breaktime that Joshua had kicked his bag into the aisle?**

- He probably didn't want to make matters worse by getting Joshua into further trouble – it would make it even harder to make up and be friends again.
- He couldn't grass on him a second time – he'd learnt his lesson.
- Shaun may have felt he deserved to take the blame as punishment for what he did to Joshua.
- Miss Atkinson may have thought Shaun was trying to push the blame unfairly onto his friend, and may well have liked him less for it.

6. **(a) Did revenge make Joshua feel good about himself?**

No – it definitely made Joshua feel bad about himself.

(b) Have you ever done something similar? How did you feel?

(Personal responses required.)

7. *Has someone ever taken revenge on you? How did it make you feel?*
(Personal responses required.)

8. *Was there a better way of Joshua getting his own back?*

- If some sort of revenge is required, being ignored is very hurtful and it was working successfully – Shaun was very unhappy about being ignored.
- He could have told Shaun's parents what Shaun had done – but that wouldn't put him in a good light for telling on Shaun.
- He could have called him a grass to his face and confronted him about the whole situation instead of immediately shunning him. He may have understood Shaun's motives better.

9. *If Joshua wanted Shaun to stay his friend could he have shown how hurt he was in some other way?*

- He could have told Shaun off privately – then less damage would have been done.
- He could have told Shaun about the trouble he'd got into with his Dad and made him apologise again.
- He could sit down with him and talk it over and make new ground rules for their relationship. ('If you ever do that again I'll…') However, that's very hard to do when you're hurting and feeling resentful, and it's a mature step to take. Joshua is very young.

10. *Shaun blamed Joshua for him getting into trouble and not getting his bike for his birthday. Was this fair?*

Yes: Because it was Joshua's actions that prompted Miss Atkinson to give Shaun a detention. If a detention had been given just because Shaun had forgotten his pencil case then it would have been Shaun's responsibility.

No: Joshua did not know that Shaun's dad had promised him a bike if he kept out of trouble so cannot be responsible for that.

STORY 3: Goodbye Shaun

'Here again?' Jabo asked the white boy standing outside the sweet shop. 'Haven't you got a home to go to?' The boy didn't answer. 'What's your name?'

'Shaun.'

'Shaun,' Jabo mimicked. 'Isn't that cute. Hear that, Martha?' Jabo's arm was draped over Martha's shoulder. 'Why don't you come with us and grab a piece of the action?' Jabo challenged.

'No thanks. I'm going home.' It wasn't true. Usually, he spent Wednesdays at his friend Joshua's house but they had fallen out and he was too ashamed to tell his parents. So he hung around after school until it was the usual time to show his face.

'Come on, man. Live a little,' Jabo invited. 'Two kids from your year are going. Shane and Rachel.' Shaun knew who they were but hadn't ever talked to them. They were in a different class to him. 'Right. Let's go.' Jabo took it for granted that Shaun would follow. There was a gate in an alley at the back of a garden, and Jabo climbed over the fence to open it for them. 'In here.' He motioned to an old shed once they were through. Shane and Rachel arrived at the same time. 'Got the stuff?' Jabo asked them. Shane lifted up a plastic carrier bag. Shaun wondered what was inside it.

'Whose shed is this?' Shaun asked nervously. He wished he hadn't come but it was too late to back out now.

'Who cares?' Rachel answered. 'No one ever comes here. That's all that matters.'

'Why?' Shaun asked.

'Questions, questions,' Jabo laughed. 'Anyone would think you were straight out of nursery.' They all laughed and Shaun shut up. 'Here's for some fun. Try it, you'll probably like it,' Jabo told Shaun.

They were sitting on the floor in a rough circle. Several clear plastic bags were produced with two aerosol cans. Shaun suddenly felt very frightened. He wanted to go. 'I've just remembered. I promised I'd phone my mum. She'll be worried sick. I've got to go.' Shaun reached the door, but not before Rachel.

'Scared, little boy?' she taunted.

Shaun gulped. 'Course not.'

'Then sit down and join us. It'll make you feel better. Honest.' Rachel smiled and Shaun realised she was very pretty. He sat down. He knew they wouldn't let him go. He'd have to sit it out and hope that they finished soon.

Jabo was sniffing hard into a plastic bag with Martha. 'Look, this is a mug's game,' Shaun told them. 'You can get yourself killed. Or brain-damaged or something. It's like glue-sniffing.'

'Get real, will you?' Shane said impatiently. 'We've done it loads of times and we're all right. It's only the oldies trying to scare you off.' Jabo and Martha rolled over on the floor giggling. 'See?' Shane said. 'It's fun.'

Rachel handed Shaun a can and a bag. 'Try it,' she challenged. Shaun looked at Jabo and Martha doubtfully. They seemed OK, just rather jolly. Rachel filled the bag for him and put it to his face, smiling. Shaun decided it wouldn't hurt. Not just the once. He sniffed really hard, wanting to show them he wasn't scared. He was still sniffing as he fell to the floor. Shane bent over Shaun, who was lying still.

'He's dead,' Shane croaked.

'Don't fool around, Shane. It's not funny,' Rachel told him. Jabo and Martha were laughing.

'He's dead I tell you!' Shane screamed.

Jabo came to his senses. 'Let's split. Fast.'

It was two days before the police found Shaun. The verdict was death by misadventure.

Discussion Sheet 3: Goodbye Shaun

1. (a) What should Shaun have done when Jabo invited him to join them?

    (b) Would you have been afraid of losing face if someone you didn't know well challenged you like Jabo did Shaun?

2. Was it a good idea for Shaun to hang around with nowhere in particular to go? Would it have been better if he was with one of his friends?

3. Would you be too afraid or ashamed to tell your parents or guardians about breaking up with a friend? What lengths would you go to, to hide a disagreement?

4. What would you have told Shaun to do once he'd arrived at the shed and decided he didn't like it? Or was it too late for him to get away?

5. Have you ever wanted to try, or have you already tried, something that an adult has told you not to or is dangerous? If so, what was it?

6. (a) Just because you can buy certain products easily, does it mean that they are safe?

    (b) What would you say to a younger brother or sister if you saw them playing with a spray can?

7. (a) What do you know about solvent, drug or alcohol abuse?

    (b) Why do people sniff solvents if they are so dangerous?

8. Was Shaun just very unlucky, or could you yourself die using solvents?

9. (a) Who was responsible for Shaun's death?

    (b) Did Jabo, Martha, Rachel and Shane do the right thing by running away and keeping quiet about what had happened?

    (c) If not, what should they have done? (Or, what would you have done if you were one of the group?)

10. If you come across someone sniffing solvents, what should you do?

Leader Sheet 3: Goodbye Shaun

1. **(a) What should Shaun have done when Jabo invited him to join them?**

   He should have refused. He didn't know the others at all – they hadn't even known his name and they made fun of him ('white boy'). However, he was too desperate to cover up about his falling out with Joshua and decided it would fill his time.

   (b) Would you have been afraid to lose face if someone you didn't know well challenged you like Jabo did Shaun?

   (Personal response required.)

2. **Was it a good idea for Shaun to hang around with nowhere in particular to go? Would it have been better if he was with one of his friends?**

   Hanging around aimlessly makes you stand out and you become an ideal target as a victim of any kind. Being with one of his friends would have been much safer. However, at that time, Shaun didn't seem to have any friends. A shame he wasn't brave enough to tell the whole thing to his parents.

3. **Would you be too afraid or ashamed to tell your parents or guardians about breaking up with a friend? What lengths would you go to, to hide a disagreement?**

   (Personal responses required.)

4. **What would you have told Shaun to do once he'd arrived at the shed and decided he didn't like it? Or was it too late for him to get away?**

   He should have run for it, ignoring the taunts. If he didn't like it before he was in the shed, he definitely wouldn't feel comfortable inside it, trapped with the others. His pride stopped him from getting away – he was worried about being laughed at then, and at school afterwards. But it wasn't too late – they might have let him go. They hadn't forced him to go with them and seemed very relaxed about what they were doing.

5. *Have you ever wanted to try, or have you already tried, something that an adult has told you not to or is dangerous? If so, what was it?*

(Personal responses required.)

6. (a) *Just because you can buy certain products easily, does it mean that they are safe?*

Everyday products are not all safe, as the story has shown.

(b) *What would you say to a younger brother or sister if you saw them playing with a spray can?*

You could explain the dangers – if you were aware of them yourself.

7. (a) *What do you know about solvent, drug or alcohol abuse?*

Solvents:

They work as aerosol propellants for spray paints, hair lacquer, lighter fuel and deodorants. They are also used in glues, paints, paint-strippers, lacquers, petrol and cleaning fluids.

- Long-term exposure can cause (depending on what's been used) permanent liver and kidney damage, blood and liver disorders, nerve damage leading to numbness and tremor and brain damage.

- Regular use of solvents can lead to pallor, fatigue and forgetfulness, whereas heavy use can lead to weight loss, depression and a general deterioration of health.

- The signs of abuse include a chemical smell on the breath, traces of the substance on the body or clothes, unusual redness around the eyes, nose and mouth and a persistent cough. The majority of abusers are adolescents.

Drugs:

People take illegal drugs because of the effects the drugs have and because they are curious as to how they might feel. Illegal drugs are risky to take because they are dangerous and may be contaminated with other chemicals that can cause harm and their level of purity is unknown. As users' tolerance increases with habitual drug-taking, they need to take more to get the same effect, so if they suddenly get a very pure sample, the dose of the actual drug they receive can cause an overdose. When injecting, users risk catching HIV or hepatitis from using contaminated needles. It is easy to become either psychologically dependent on illegal drugs (the user feels unable to cope without it) or physically dependent (the user suffers withdrawal symptoms when he or she stops taking the drug).

There are four groups of drugs:

1. Stimulants (these increase brain activity): anabolic steroids, cocaine, crack, ecstasy, poppers, speed (amphetamines) and tobacco.

2. Depressants (these reduce brain activity): aerosols, alcohol, gases, glues, tranquillisers.

3. Hallucinogens (these distort the way users hear and see things): cannabis, ketamine, LSD, magic mushrooms.

4. Analgesics (these have a pain-killing effect): heroin.

Risks with drug-taking:

- The user can get very drowsy with heroin, tranquillisers, gases, glues and aerosols.

- The user can get tense and panic with ecstasy, LSD, magic mushrooms and speed.

- The user can get too hot and dehydrate with ecstasy and speed (the drugs affect the body's temperature control).

- The user can become unconscious with alcohol, gases, glues, aerosols, heroin, poppers, tranquillisers and (with some people) ecstasy.

- LSD can give a different trip every time and is unpredictable. It can also be responsible for flashbacks – sudden memories of previous trips, even years after taking the drug. This can be very dangerous if, for example, the person is driving at the time.

- Mixing alcohol with drugs can be fatal.

Possessing or supplying drugs is illegal. Class A drugs bring about the heaviest fines and convictions.

- Class A: cocaine, crack, ecstasy, heroin, LSD, magic mushrooms (if prepared for use), speed (if prepared for injection).

- Class B: cannabis, speed.

- Class C: anabolic steroids, tranquillisers.

- Some other drugs can be legally possessed but it is an offence to supply them.

Alcohol:

Long-term heavy use of alcohol can lead to dependence and health problems such as heart and circulatory disorders, liver disease, ulcers and brain damage. It impairs judgement, making accidents more likely, and reduces inhibitions so there is greater risk of having unprotected sex. (Alcohol is looked at in more detail in *Story 19: I Don't Remember.*)

(b) Why do people sniff solvents if they are so dangerous?

They are sniffed because of (illegal) drug-like effects: light-headedness, dizziness, confusion, drowsiness and loss of co-ordination. Sometimes, with larger doses, the sniffer experiences disorientation, hallucinations and loss of consciousness.

8. Was Shaun just very unlucky, or could you yourself die using solvents?

- Solvent abuse can cause heart failure, even on the first attempt. The Department of Health has reported that about one third of solvent deaths occur on what was probably the person's first attempt at sniffing.

- Aerosol gases, butane gas and cleaning fluids can cause heart failure and death.

- Aerosol and butane gas can cause death from suffocation by sudden freezing of the air passages. Butane gas can ignite in the mouth.

- Deodorants and paints coat the lungs and can suffocate you.

- You can suffocate if you inhale using a plastic bag. The risk increases if you vomit while you are inhaling from a plastic bag. (The solvent can make you feel sick and you might actually be sick. It can also give you headaches.)

- You can die even if you have been sniffing regularly. If you are startled under the influence of solvents, your heart might stop. Or you might have an accident while under the influence of the solvent because you don't know what you are doing.

- The Department of Health has reported that one in ten secondary pupils will try sniffing solvents.

9. (a) Who was responsible for Shaun's death?

Rachel was directly responsible for Shaun's death as she had handed him the solvent to sniff and persuaded him to do it. However, morally Jabo, Martha, and Shane are also responsible as they provided the solvent and the environment in which to do it, and goaded him into trying. Shaun himself also should take some responsibility. He wasn't forcibly held down and made to inhale. However, the others had made it difficult for him to refuse.

(b) Did Jabo, Martha, Rachel and Shane do the right thing by running away and keeping quiet about what had happened?

Not by his parents – or by Shaun himself. His parents would have been worried sick as it was two days before Shaun was found. They had probably imagined him abducted and horribly murdered. It also wasn't respectful to Shaun to leave his body to rot in a cold, dark and unfriendly place, away from his loved ones. He had died at their hands and they'd just run off and left him. They should have taken responsibility for what had happened.

(c) If not, what should they have done? (Or, what would you have done if you were one of the group?)

Two of them could have stayed with Shaun's body while the others went to call for an ambulance. However, if that was too hard for them, they could have phoned the ambulance anonymously so that Shaun wouldn't have been left for two days.

10. If you come across someone sniffing solvents, what should you do?

- Don't scare the person in any way, especially by shouting, as this can make his or her heart stop.
- You should not interrupt the person but go and tell a responsible adult.
- If the person has collapsed, you must get medical help.
- If the person's parents or guardians are nearby, you could tell them but impress upon them first that they must not frighten their child as it could make his or her heart stop.

STORY 4: Extortion!

'Have you borrowed any money from me?' Mrs Richards asked her husband.

'No. Is some missing again?'

'Five pounds. I'm sure of it this time,' she said, checking her purse. 'I'm going to have it out with Hannah.'

Hannah was busy doing her homework. 'Did you take five pounds from my purse, Hannah?' her mother asked.

'No.'

'Empty your pockets, school bag and blazer, please. Money doesn't walk by itself, Hannah.' Hannah dutifully emptied her pockets and bag. 'You've missed the front pouch of your bag,' Mrs Edwards informed her, rather sternly.

Hannah reluctantly produced a five-pound note. 'Explain,' her mother said harshly, turning pale at the thought of her daughter being a thief. Hannah burst into tears and the story came pouring out. Her mother was shocked. 'I'm going to demand that the school does something. How much money has this Rachel had out of you altogether?'

'Thirty pounds,' Hannah admitted. She had been too scared and ashamed to admit to her parents what had been going on.

Mr Eleftheriou sat opposite Rachel in his office. Her mother had already been called and was on her way. His Deputy Head of Year, Miss O'Connor, was also present. 'Extortion is extremely serious, Rachel. So far, I've discovered two other girls who have been giving you money because you threatened them. When your mother arrives we shall consult with the Headteacher over this and decide whether you are to be expelled. What did you want the money for?'

Rachel didn't answer. Mr Eleftheriou noticed she had a rash around her mouth and nose. It didn't look like acne to him. 'I think it's time to empty your bag, Rachel. If you don't oblige, Miss O'Connor can do it for you.' The bag contained only books. 'Let's look in your locker.'

As the locker door opened, they saw a carrier bag. Inside were two spray cans. 'Well, well, well,' Mr Eleftheriou said grimly. 'The plot thickens.'

Mr Eleftheriou made a call to the local police. 'We have a Miss Rachel Somers here who may be able to help you with your enquiries in respect of Shaun Robinson. It appears she has glue-sniffer's rash and is in possession of two canisters.'

Mr Eleftheriou informed Rachel that two officers were coming to interview her and would arrange for a medical opinion on her rash and a blood sample if the doctor thought it necessary.

'So what if I've tried sniffing? There's no law against it and you can't prove anything about this Shaun Robinson,' Rachel spat out viciously.

'You'd be surprised what the police can do. Enough calling cards were left where Shaun died from what I gather. They obtained good fingerprints from the cans. They just needed a lead as to where to start looking. If it turns out you were with Shaun when he died you will be in more trouble than you could ever imagine possible. It won't look good that you left him without getting help.'

'I want to go to the toilet,' Rachel told him coldly.

'Certainly. We'll escort you and Miss O'Connor will go in with you. I'm not having you free to communicate with any of your so-called mates and I'm not letting you run off without seeing the police first. Do you still need to go?'

Rachel swore at him.

'The way I see it, the school will be pleased to get rid of your corrupting influence. And your friends can go with you if any of their prints match up. I'm sure the Headteacher will agree. He takes a dim view of solvent abuse and extortion. You are well on the road to nowhere, Rachel Somers.'

Discussion Sheet 4: Extortion!

1. What is extortion?

2. (a) What sort of person do you think an extortionist is?

   (b) Why do extortionists use threats to get money?

   (c) What drives them to it?

3. Would you steal to pay an extortionist? Or would you risk the threats and tell a responsible adult? Or just tell your best friend?

4. What would you do if you knew that your best friend was threatened and had been told to give someone money?

5. What do you think might happen if an extortionist is allowed to get away with his or her crimes? Will he or she continue to terrorise people even after leaving school?

6. (a) Have you ever forced someone to give you something using threats or emotional blackmail ('If you don't give me that, I'll tell about…')?

    (b) If so, how did it make you feel?

    (c) Were you proud of your behaviour?

7. Because Rachel was getting money from other pupils, she was able to keep buying solvents. If she had been found out sooner she may have had help sooner for her problem. What sort of help do you think Rachel needs?

8. Why do you think Rachel and her friends kept quiet about their involvement with Shaun when he died?

9. Do you hate or pity Rachel? Why?

10. Do you think she'd ever forget her part in Shaun's death?

Leader Sheet 4: Extortion!

1. ***What is extortion?***
   It is using threats to get people to give you money and is a form of bullying.

2. ***(a) What sort of person do you think an extortionist is?***
   An extortionist is:

   - a bully
   - someone who only cares about him or herself
   - someone who doesn't think criminal activity is wrong
   - someone who doesn't care what other people think of him or her
   - someone who likes to have power over people and see them do his or her bidding
   - someone who wants the good things in life to come easily without having to work for them.

   (b) Why do extortionists use threats to get money?
   Extortionists use threats to get money probably because they want it quickly, and are not prepared to earn it. If they don't threaten the person they want to take it from, the person won't give it.

   (c) What drives them to it?
   - They may desperately want the money to support addictive habits.
   - They may feel a need to control others – they may be abused at home and take out their frustration on those emotionally weaker than themselves.
   - They may do it for entertainment.
   - They may do it because it's about all they are good at and want to prove to others there is something they do well.
   - They may do it to look powerful in front of their friends.

3. ***Would you steal to pay an extortionist? Or would you risk the threats and tell a responsible adult? Or just tell your best friend?***
   (Personal responses required.)

4. *What would you do if you knew that your best friend was threatened and had been told to give someone money?*

(Personal response required.)

5. *What do you think might happen if an extortionist is allowed to get away with his or her crimes? Will he or she continue to terrorise people even after leaving school?*

Once people know they can get away with criminal or bullying activities, it is unlikely that they will stop of their own accord. Rachel's behaviour has been anti-social – she hasn't cared about the feelings of the people around her or thought of the agonies Shaun's family must have gone through for those two days he was missing. She also hadn't cared about breaking school rules or using other people's property. She probably will continue to terrorise people – if she gets the chance.

6. *(a) Have you ever forced someone to give you something using threats or emotional blackmail ('If you don't give me that, I'll tell about...')?*

(Personal response required.)

(b) If so, how did it make you feel?

Suggestions: clever, guilty, in control, mean, powerful, resourceful, strong, worried about the shame of being caught.

(c) Were you proud of your behaviour?

(Personal response required.)

7. *Because Rachel was getting money from other pupils, she was able to keep buying solvents. If she had been found out sooner she may have had help sooner for her problem. What sort of help do you think Rachel needs?*

- She may be addicted to solvents and may need help to fight it.
- She may need counselling to find out why she started to sniff solvents in the first place.
- She may need counselling to help her psychological dependence on solvents (she may feel she cannot cope with life without them).

8. Why do you think Rachel and her friends kept quiet about their involvement with Shaun when he died?

- They did not want to get into trouble.
- They didn't want anyone to know that they sniff solvents.
- They were very scared of what might happen to them and how people would react towards them if they did know.

9. Do you hate or pity Rachel? Why?

Hate: She had no right to try to force someone to do something dangerous.

She was a coward for running away when Shaun died.

She didn't mend her ways after the shock of his death and the part in it that she'd played. She was still sniffing glue and extorting money to pay for it.

Pity: She's a mixed-up girl.

She has jeopardised her future. She may be expelled and have what she did on her school record. She may also end up with a police record.

10. Do you think she'd ever forget her part in Shaun's death?

- Rachel didn't seem very sorry about Shaun's death – when she was questioned about it by Mr Eleftheriou, she didn't break down and cry. She seems quite a hardened character. Perhaps she'll look back in several years' time and then be more regretful – when she has children of her own and understands the agonies of being a parent.
- Suffering expulsion and perhaps having to appear in court will stay with her. These may have long-term consequences in how she is treated in her next school and how good a reference she will get when she wants to leave. Having something on her police record might affect her future career.
- People arond her may not allow her to forget. All her family and neighbours will know about her as the event is likely to be reported in the local papers and they will probably keep reminding her about it. She may feel she has to leave the area and start afresh as soon as she gets the opportunity.

STORY 5: 'Atch Out!!

'This is Robert Nyinaku. He's joining your class from today,' Mrs Price announced to her form. 'I'm seating him next to Sally.' There was a hush as Robert sat down. He was in Shaun's place and no one else had sat there since his death. Robert didn't know why people kept giving him angry looks but it made him nervous. And his stammer always got worse when he was nervous.

When the bell went for the first lesson, Robert followed without anyone talking to him.

'Are you new?' Mr Khan asked Robert as he entered the history class.

'Yyes sssir.' The class began to snigger. 'Name?' Mr Khan asked, ignoring the class.

'Rrrobert Nnnnyinnaku,' Robert managed painfully. He felt as though he could die of embarrassment. What a way to begin his first day. The class was laughing openly now, the infection having spread.

'Sit next to Shirley Prasad, please.' Mr Khan pointed to a vacant chair.

'Hi, Rrrrobbbert,' Shirley joked. The class roared with laughter this time and Robert looked as though he was about to burst into tears.

'I've had enough of your humour for one day, Year Eight,' Mr Khan told them angrily. 'Your jokes are unacceptable to me and most definitely unacceptable to Robert. I am appalled at your lack of feeling. All of you here have something that is individual to you and you should be glad that you are all so different.

'Joshua, you were laughing. How would you feel in an all-white school where people laughed at you because you were black? And you, Sally, would look out of place in a black community. Malika, no one laughs at you for always having your head covered. All of you would have somewhere where you would be out of place. If Robert were in a class full of stammerers he would not be out of place. I demand you have the same respect for him as you expect to have from others. Have I made myself clear?'

'Yes, sir,' the class obediently replied in unison. However, Robert was gently ridiculed throughout the day and the class tried to hide their laughter each time Robert was asked a question.

At the end of the day, Robert left the school gates at the same time as Joshua. Joshua was going to ask Robert where he lived but decided against it as it took Robert so long to answer. He was still hurting from losing Shaun and felt guilty about making a new friend. Shaun might think he'd deserted his memory. Deep in thought, Joshua said goodbye to Robert before crossing the road. He forgot to look.

'Atch out!!' Robert cried as he saw the oncoming car.

Joshua stopped just in time to see the pale face of the driver go past. He'd almost been run over! Feeling weak, he sat down by the fence. Robert had saved him. He should have paid attention to where he was going.

'Are yyou all rright?' asked Robert.

Joshua nodded. 'What was it you shouted?'

'Atch out.' Robert repeated. 'If I'd ttried wwwatch out I'd have ggot stuck on the dddoubble u and then you wouldn't have heard.'

'That was really clever of you. D'you want to be friends?' Joshua asked shyly.

'Ttthank yyou. I had to mmove from mmy last school as mmy Mmum died. I'm living with mmy Ddad now.' Robert told him.

'One of my best friends died too,' Joshua said. He had been cruel to Robert when underneath, Robert had the same feelings as everyone else. He was surprised that Robert didn't hate him for laughing.

Discussion Sheet 5: 'Atch Out!!

1. (a) Has someone you know died recently? How close were you?

   (b) How did you feel? (Or, how do you think someone might feel?)

2. (a) How do you think Joshua felt about Robert sitting in Shaun's place?

   (b) What could he have said to himself to help him try not to mind?

   (c) Was Mrs Price right to seat Robert there?

3. Do you know anyone who has a slight disability such as stammering or is partially sighted or profoundly deaf? Do you treat them with impatience or with understanding? Do you behave differently towards them in ways not connected with their disability? (For example, do you treat them as though they were stupid? Or talk extra loud when there's nothing wrong with their hearing?)

4. (a) How does Robert feel about having a stammer?

   (b) If you developed a stammer, would your friends treat you differently?

5. Do you think it was funny that Robert was laughed at, or do you think it was wrong of the class to laugh? Why?

6. How would you have reacted in Joshua's class? (If the rest of the class were laughing, would you have joined in?)

7. What message was Mr Khan trying to get across about being different?

8. Why didn't Joshua want to make friends with Robert when they first met?

9. Why do you think Robert didn't hate Joshua for laughing with the rest of the class?

10. What important issue was this story getting at? (Look at the last paragraph.)

Leader Sheet 5: 'Atch Out!!

1. **(a) Has someone you know died recently? How close were you?**
(Personal response required.)

   (b) How did you feel? (Or, how do you think someone might feel?)
   - Angry – that the person has left you to cope on your own.
   - Angry – that you did not have a chance to say all you wanted to.
   - Depressed – you feel that there is no point to life without the person who has died.
   - Disbelief – that the person has really gone.
   - Guilt – for still being alive when the other person is dead.
   - Guilt – for the wrongs you did to the person and for not putting them right.
   - Regret – that the person's life had ended 'before time' or before the person had had a chance to fulfil his or her dreams, living life to the full.
   - Regret – that you will have to make your way without this person, unable to share new experiences.
   - Sad – you miss the person.
   - Scared – of what the future might hold and of being left alone.
   - Shocked and numbed – you don't know how you feel and nothing seems real.

2. **(a) How do you think Joshua felt about Robert sitting in Shaun's place?**
   - Angry – the teacher shouldn't have told Robert to sit there; it was insensitive of her.
   - Resentful – Robert had no right to sit in Shaun's place.
   - Sad – it was another sign that Shaun wasn't ever coming back.

   (b) What could he have said to himself to help him try not to mind?
   - 'Life goes on.'

- 'I can't mourn Shaun in such an intense way forever.'
- 'Robert hasn't hurt my feelings deliberately and probably doesn't even know about Shaun. In fact, if he did know, he probably wouldn't want to sit there either.'

(c) Was Mrs Price right to seat Robert there?

Yes:

- If Shaun's place was deliberately left empty, it would seem as though he still 'owned' his place and that he was still sitting there.
- By getting Robert to sit there, the class would soon think of it as Robert's place rather than Shaun's.
- It was showing the class that life must go on and things had to move forward.
- It must have been terrible for Sally sitting next to an empty space – seating Robert there would have helped her.

No:

- It was insensitive of her to seat Robert in Shaun's place so soon after his death – both for the class, mourning Shaun's loss, and for Robert, who knew nothing about Shaun's death. If he'd known, he wouldn't have wanted to sit there.

Note: No mention was made in the story whether there were any other empty seats. So it is not known whether this was a deliberate move by Mrs Price or an unavoidable one. Another way out of this situation would have been to mix up the entire class, rearranging the chairs and tables so that no one was sitting in their usual place. Then Robert would not have been usurping Shaun's place.

3. *Do you know anyone who has a slight disability such as stammering or is partially sighted or profoundly deaf? Do you treat them with impatience or with understanding? Do you behave differently towards them in ways not connected with their disability? (For example, do you treat them as though they were stupid? Or talk extra loud when there's nothing wrong with their hearing?)*

(Personal responses required.)

4. **(a) How does Robert feel about having a stammer?**

   - Robert must feel extremely self-conscious.
   - He probably wants to crawl into the floor with embarrassment every time a teacher asks him a question in front of the class.
   - He probably dreads meeting new people, as the first thing they will notice is his speech and then they may not look beyond it to the person inside.
   - He must dread being teased.

   (b) If you developed a stammer, would your friends treat you differently?

   Children and adolescents are often cruel – they probably would make fun of you if you had a stammer.

5. **Do you think it was funny that Robert was laughed at or do you think it was wrong of the class to laugh? Why?**

   It was wrong of the class to laugh at Robert because they publicly humiliated him. They hadn't thought of how it must feel to be the only one starting a new school in the middle of term, when everyone else was familiar with the place and teachers, and had friends. They probably understood about racism and sexism and didn't make racist and sexist remarks (Mr Khan reminded them of what he thought they already knew) but they hadn't extended this education to people with disabilities.

6. **How would you have reacted in Joshua's class? (If the rest of the class were laughing, would you have joined in?)**

   (Personal response required.)

   (It's very tempting to join in with the pack. When you might not make fun of someone on your own, it's a different matter in the safety of a crowd.)

7. **What message was Mr Khan trying to get across about being different?**

   You should accept others as you find them, without being judgemental or only seeing superficial things. He wanted his pupils to think for themselves – they had a right not to be singled out because of race, and Robert had a right not to be singled out because of his disability.

8. **Why didn't Joshua want to make friends with Robert when they first met?**

- He was hurting from losing Shaun.

- He couldn't bear that someone else was in Shaun's place.

- He felt guilty about Shaun's death. (Shaun would have been at Joshua's house for tea the night he died if they hadn't fallen out with each other.)

- He didn't want Shaun to think he'd forgotten about him so soon.

- It took Robert so long to say something, Joshua couldn't be bothered to give him the time.

9. **Why do you think Robert didn't hate Joshua for laughing with the rest of the class?**

- He was probably used to ridicule and understood the others were behaving like sheep – not thinking for themselves but joining in with the 'flock'.

- He couldn't afford to be too picky – he didn't have any friends at this school.

- He was hurting because his mum had died. He was desperate to make any kind of friend.

10. **What important issue was this story getting at? (Look at the last paragraph.)**

You shouldn't make snap judgements and dismiss people so easily for not being suitable as a friend. Like people, friendships come in all forms. If you only take the trouble to look, you'll probably find you have more in common with a person than you think.

STORY 6: Science Test!

'Preeti, I wanted to see you before the exam papers were handed back this afternoon,' Miss Atkinson told her. Two days ago, Preeti had sat the end-of-term science exam.

'Could you explain how you and Sally have virtually identical answers?' Preeti didn't answer. 'Did you copy off Sally, Preeti?' Miss Atkinson asked sternly.

'No, Miss.'

'Then how do you account for having the same answers? Are you saying that Sally copied off you?'

'I don't know if she did, Miss. I was busy doing the paper.'

Miss Atkinson hated these interviews. 'Preeti, when two people manage to get the same *wrong* answers, alarm bells start to ring. This sort of thing does not happen by coincidence. And Sally sat in front of you in the exam. Now, did you copy from her?'

'No!' Preeti cried out.

Miss Atkinson showed Preeti her paper and compared it to Sally's, pointing out all the improbable coincidences of their answers. 'You are making it harder on yourself and Sally by not telling me what went on. Who copied from whom?' Preeti remained silent. 'You realise that both you and Sally will have nought for the science test? The rules of cheating were made clear?' Miss Atkinson asked. Preeti nodded. 'Now if one of you doesn't own up I'll have no choice but to write on both your reports that you cheated. The person who allowed it to happen is just as much at fault as the one who copied – but the one who copied should never have started it in the first place. It is a very serious matter and an ugly one. I can see both of you getting into a great deal of trouble with your parents.'

'It was me, Miss,' Preeti admitted.

'Now why didn't you save us the unpleasantness and admit it sooner? If you do something wrong, be big and own up straight away. Don't let others take the blame.' Miss Atkinson was disappointed in Preeti. 'Why did you do it? Hadn't you learnt the work?'

'I had but I found it hard. My dad likes me to do well.'

'And you hadn't wanted to disappoint him?' Miss Atkinson asked sympathetically. Preeti nodded. 'Would your dad have wanted you to have got good marks through cheating?'

'No, Miss,' Preeti answered miserably.

'And now you have no marks at all. You'd have done better on your own. What will your dad say?'

Preeti swallowed, hard. 'I don't know. He wants me to be a doctor.'

'Has your dad actually said that?'

'No, but I know it's what he wants from what he says. My uncle's a doctor.'

'Preeti, I think it will be a good idea if I see your dad one afternoon. It's too soon to be thinking of a career for you and maybe he doesn't realise he's put pressure on you to do well. All anyone can ask is that you do your best.' Miss Atkinson paused. 'I'm disappointed that you resorted to cheating. If you've got a problem, you should talk it over with your parents or a teacher you feel you can trust. It will have to go on your school record that you cheated.

'I've lost trust in you, Preeti. I will keep a close eye on every piece of homework and separate you and Sally in all exams. You'll find that once you've lost someone's trust it's extremely hard to get it back. Getting nought is only going to be one of your problems! Now, go and apologise to Sally.'

Discussion Sheet 6: Science Test!

1. Have you ever cheated in an exam? If so, why?

2. Did you get found out? If so, what happened? Did it stop you from doing it again?

3. (a) Is copying someone else's homework and presenting it as your own the same as cheating?

    (b) What about in real life – if you steal someone else's ideas, writings or inventions it is known as plagiarism. Is that cheating?

4. (a) Have you ever helped anyone to cheat – not just in exams? If you have, why did you do it?

(b) Did you regret it afterwards?

5. (a) Is it friendly to expect someone to let you copy his or her work?

   (b) Adolescents tend to be in a hurry to grow up. Isn't being responsible for themselves a necessary part of that?

6. Do you agree with Miss Atkinson that the person who allows the cheating to go ahead is equally at fault?

7. What happens in external exams (for example, GCSEs) when examiners notice similar coincidences?

8. Why do you think Miss Atkinson was so harsh with Preeti?

9. What do you think of cheating in general? That it's wrong, whatever the reasons? That it's fine as long as you don't get caught? Or that it's the only way for you to get on?

10. Is it fair to get recognition for something you don't deserve? Is it worth it?

Leader Sheet 6: Science Test!

1. **Have you ever cheated in an exam? If so, why?**
    - Because of parental pressure.
    - Because you want to be better than you are.
    - To hide the fact that you didn't revise.
    - To hide the fact that you don't understand the work.

2. **Did you get found out? If so, what happened? Did it stop you from doing it again?**
    (Personal responses required.)

3. **(a) Is copying someone else's homework and presenting it as your own the same as cheating?**
    Yes, copying anything for which you get the credit is cheating.

    (b) What about in real life – if you steal someone else's ideas, writings or inventions it is known as plagiarism. Is that cheating?
    If you plagiarise someone else's work it is cheating. For example, some high street shops have copied designer clothes, and have made money from other people's investments in designers and in developing new ideas. They have profited from others' hard work.

4. **(a) Have you ever helped anyone to cheat – not just in exams? If you have, why did you do it?**
    - To gain friendship.
    - Because you were frightened of the person.
    - Because the person was your friend.
    - Because you felt sorry for the person.

    (b) Did you regret it afterwards?
    (Personal response required.)

5. **(a) Is it friendly to expect someone to let you copy his or her work?**

    Yes: They can copy yours any time. Friends should help each other out. Even adults ask help from one another. It's what people do.

    No: But it's very hard to refuse and it helps you not get into trouble.

    (b) Adolescents tend to be in a hurry to grow up. Isn't being responsible for themselves a necessary part of that?

    Yes. If you put in all the work, why should others benefit from it? Copying doesn't help them in the long run, when it's the external exams. And it doesn't help them understand the work, so they'll get behind without the teacher knowing they need extra help. Eventually they will have to stand on their own two feet so the sooner they learn, the better at it they will be.

6. **Do you agree with Miss Atkinson that the person who allows the cheating to go ahead is equally at fault?**

    Theoretically, yes – both are at fault. But allowing someone to read your work is a passive acceptance, whereas actually straining to read another's work in a test, or asking to copy the homework, is active, calculated behaviour.

7. **What happens in external exams (for example, GCSEs) when examiners notice similar coincidences?**

    Similar wrong answers that are peculiar to two papers alert external examiners to the possibility of cheating having occurred. They then check the seating plans for that exam, supplied by your school. If you are caught cheating, the invigilator will have to submit a report and the incident will be investigated. You risk having your paper cancelled. And if you were knowingly helped by another candidate, their paper could be cancelled too.

8. **Why do you think Miss Atkinson was so harsh with Preeti?**

    So that she didn't ever copy again and didn't risk copying in the external exams, where the consequences are so much greater.

9. ***What do you think of cheating in general? That it's wrong, whatever the reasons? That it's fine as long as you don't get caught? Or that it's the only way for you to get on?***

   (Personal responses required.)

10. ***Is it fair to get recognition for something you don't deserve? Is it worth it?***

   No, it's not fair – but if you get away with it, you'll probably consider it worth it in the short term. However, assuming you don't risk cheating in the external exams, your results will then suddenly become very low and you won't achieve your predicted grades. You can't get away with copying forever.

STORY 7: *Hoi Ping Is Unhappy*

'These forms are for you to make appointments with your teachers so your parents can see them next week,' Mrs Price told her registration class.

'Are your parents coming this time, Hoi Ping?' Rajesh asked.

Hoi Ping shook his head. They were always too busy with the Take-Away. His family worked very hard and they couldn't just close down for an evening. But he really wished they could come and see his teachers and his school.

As the week drew on, Hoi Ping became more miserable. Some pupils were so naughty their parents were always up at the school. 'It's not fair,' he thought angrily as he was walked across the schoolyard from one lesson to the next.

Hoi Ping picked up a stone and threw it furiously at a wall, venting his anger and frustration. But it missed and went straight through a window, smashing the pane of glass!

Mrs Ng was called up to the school the same day. Hoi Ping was normally such a good boy she just couldn't believe what he'd done. Hoi Ping sat opposite her, studying the ground.

'Have you any idea of what might be troubling him?' Mr Eleftheriou, the Head of Year, asked.

Mrs Ng shook her head. Surely her son wasn't turning into a hooligan? They'd tried so hard to bring him up well, to teach him the difference between right and wrong.

'Hoi Ping, can you tell us why you did it?' Hoi Ping shook his head, keeping his eyes low. 'I've heard that you've been very upset about parents' evening. Apparently, you feel left out because no one comes. Is that why you were angry and threw the stone?'

Hoi Ping nodded. Rajesh must have stuck up for him. 'I didn't throw it at the window. It was an accident.'

Mrs Ng started to cry. 'It's my fault, I don't have enough time for him – there is always so much to do.'

'Why didn't you tell your mother how you felt, Hoi Ping?'

'We all work so hard. I didn't want to make her feel bad about it,' Hoi Ping replied.

'But that made you feel very bad, no?' Mr Eleftheriou said.

'I had no idea,' Mrs Ng sniffed. 'If only you'd said how much you wanted it we could have worked something out, I'm sure.'

'I'm sorry,' Hoi Ping told his mother.

'We do need to punish Hoi Ping,' Mr Eleftheriou said, after a pause. 'He could have blinded someone or knocked them out. Glass splinters were found all over the room. He was lucky the classroom was empty at the time. I'm suspending him for the rest of the day.

'Maybe you will be able to talk over any problems before he comes back tomorrow. At least we understand why he did it and I am sure he won't do it again.'

Hoi Ping shook his head vigorously.

'Perhaps Hoi Ping could decide which teachers he'd particularly like you to see and ask them if they are happy to make an appointment one lunchtime, when you're not so busy at the shop?'

Mrs Ng smiled. 'Parents should be there for you, Hoi Ping, and if they're busy you must make them listen. Yes?'

Hoi Ping nodded earnestly as they left.

'How are we going to tell your father? This is no way to repay us for our hard work. We have to provide food and clothes for you both. We do it for you and Kit Ming. The shame of it!'

Hoi Ping was in for a hard time and wished he could stay at school.

Discussion Sheet 7: Hoi Ping Is Unhappy

1. Do your parents or guardians always go to parents' evenings? (Or concerts or plays that you've been in?) Do you wish they didn't or are you glad of their support? How do you feel if they rarely or never go?

2. (a) How do you think Hoi Ping felt?

   (b) Was he expecting good reports, do you think?

   (c) Why did he want a parent to be there?

3. What did Hoi Ping's parents expect from him?

4. (a) Do you think Hoi Ping's mother would have managed to go to parents' evening if she had known how upset her son was?

   (b) What must it be like to run a Take-Away?

5. Have you ever felt let down by your parents or guardians because they are so busy? Perhaps they work long hours or your mother has just had a baby – or they have too many problems of their own to take yours on board as well.

6. Have you tried to get them to listen to you? What did you do? Did it work? If not, did you try again? Or did you feel too rejected?

7. (a) What should Hoi Ping have done to let his parents know how he felt?

   (b) Was it fair on his parents to expect them somehow to know how he felt?

8. Do you have a duty to yourself to make sure you are taken seriously?

9. If your parents or guardians don't listen to you, do you automatically think it's because they don't care? If you saw the same thing happening with a younger brother or sister would you try to help them get their message across?

10. Do Hoi Ping's parents love him? Try to explain your answer.

Leader Sheet 7: Hoi Ping Is Unhappy

1. *Do your parents or guardians always go to parents' evenings? (Or concerts or plays that you've been in?) Do you wish they didn't or are you glad of their support? How do you feel if they rarely or never go?*

(Personal responses required.)

2. *(a) How do you think Hoi Ping felt?*

- Embarrassed – at being different from the rest and having to answer everyone's questions about why his parents weren't going.

- Left out – he was the only one who wasn't taking an appointment sheet for teachers to write in a consultation time, and he was the only one who wasn't talking about the coming evening and surmising what teachers might say.

- Unloved – his parents didn't care about him enough to make the effort to get to school.

(b) Was he expecting good reports, do you think?

It may have had nothing to do with expecting a good report. (But it certainly wouldn't have been a bad report because then he wouldn't have wanted them to go – judging by the fear of the trouble he's going to be in when he gets home.)

(c) Why did he want a parent to be there?

- To be like everyone else.

- To share in friends' chatter and feel a part of what was going on.

- To have it publicly recognised that his parents thought enough of him to make the effort to attend.

- He said he wanted his parents to see his teachers and his school.

3. *What did Hoi Ping's parents expect from him?*

They expect him to be 'well brought up'. That means being polite, obedient and hard-working; complying with school rules and never getting into trouble. They probably also want him to do well and have great hopes for his future.

4. (a) Do you think Hoi Ping's mother would have managed to go to parents' evening if she had known how upset her son was?

Yes. She seemed genuinely hurt that Hoi Ping hadn't told her how upset he was about her not going and she said that she would have found a way.

(b) What must it be like to run a Take-Away?

Running a Take-Away must be very hard work. They are sometimes open at lunchtimes and in the evenings until very late (usually midnight). As well as having their own housework and correspondence to deal with, Take-Away owners have to:

- buy the food for the shop
- be in regular contact with the suppliers
- keep an eye on stock and top up before they run out
- keep an eye on the use-by dates and freshness of the food
- do plenty of washing up
- keep the kitchen clean
- prepare much of the food before the shop opens (washing and slicing vegetables and meat)
- keep accounts
- pay wages
- fill in tax forms.

5. Have you ever felt let down by your parents or guardians because they are so busy? Perhaps they work long hours or your mother has just had a baby – or they have too many problems of their own to take yours on board as well.

(Personal response required.)

6. Have you tried to get them to listen to you? What did you do? Did it work? If not, did you try again? Or did you feel too rejected?

(Personal responses required.)

7. (a) What should Hoi Ping have done to let his parents know how he felt?

He should have told them he wanted to talk to them and, once he'd got their attention, explained how he felt.

(b) Was it fair on his parents to expect them somehow to know how he felt?

Hoi Ping blamed his parents but part of it was his responsibility because he can't expect them to guess all he's feeling. They should have paid him more attention, but he hadn't thought to try talking to them because they were so busy.

8. Do you have a duty to yourself to make sure you are taken seriously?

Yes. Expressing your needs and desires helps you have a high self-esteem. You have a right to make your needs known. However, people also have a right to refuse requests, but at least you'd have tried.

9. If your parents or guardians don't listen to you, do you automatically think it's because they don't care? If you saw the same thing happening with a younger brother or sister would you try to help them get their message across?

(Personal responses required.)

10. Do Hoi Ping's parents love him? Try to explain your answer.

- His mum certainly does, otherwise she would not have shown so much concern about what had happened at school and she wouldn't have cried, feeling guilty about neglecting Hoi Ping's needs.

- His father probably does too, otherwise he would not work so hard for his family. He probably wants his son to have a different life to his and feels that this is one way of contributing – giving his son a secure home without financial worries so that he has the opportunity to continue his education.

STORY 8: *It Happened One Day*

'Rajesh, you wanted to talk to me about something,' the counsellor said.

Rajesh sat silent. He didn't know where to start. He felt so stupid.

'Rajesh,' said the counsellor again, 'Mr Khan told me that you had had a talk with him, and that you agreed to come and see me.'

'Yes,' admitted Rajesh, mumbling.

'And now you don't want to talk?'

Rajesh said nothing. He did want to talk but he just couldn't get anything out.

The counsellor paused for a moment longer, and then added quietly, 'You don't look very happy. What's troubling you?'

'I feel so stupid,' blurted Rajesh, almost in tears now. The counsellor sat patiently, looking at him kindly. She let him take his time, and eventually Rajesh said, more calmly, 'I don't want to go to school.'

'What happened to make you feel like that?' the counsellor asked.

'I don't know,' Rajesh told her.

'When I talk about going to school, how do you feel?'

'Scared.'

'Have you always been scared of going to school?'

Rajesh shook his head.

'Can you remember the first time you were scared?'

Rajesh nodded.

'Tell me about it,' the counsellor asked gently.

'It was in the summer. When it was really hot. I have to travel by train to get to school and then a bus. It's often packed but I usually manage to get a seat. But this time my usual train was cancelled and we were boxed in like sardines. It was so hot I thought I was going to faint and then I thought I was going to be sick.'

'Were you?'

'No.'

'What were your thoughts the next time you had to get on the train?'

'I knew I just didn't want to get on. I thought I'd be sick or faint. It was such a horrible feeling you see.'

'How did you manage that journey? Did you faint?'

'I didn't but I nearly did. I was nearly sick too.' Rajesh twisted his hands together at the memory of that nightmare journey.

'I see. So am I right in thinking it's the journey to school that upsets you – not school itself?' Rajesh nodded. 'If I said to you that you didn't have to catch a train to get to school anymore, would that make school all right?'

'No.' Rajesh looked at his hands as they pulled at each other.

'What other things do you think about on the way to school? Does the bus journey upset you?'

'A bit,' Rajesh replied.

'Why is that less bad than the train journey?'

'It's not nearly so crowded. I can always get a seat. But I feel sick on buses too now. I often have to get off because I feel ill and then wait for the next one. But then I have to pay my fare as my bus pass isn't valid for any other stops – it only allows me to get on at the station.'

'I see.' The counsellor scribbled some notes. 'If you were told that you didn't have to travel on public transport to school, would you feel happy about attending?'

Rajesh thought for a moment and slowly shook his head. He felt embarrassed and oh so stupid. Whoever heard of someone afraid to use trains and buses to go to school?

'Is there anything in particular that makes you uneasy? Is every school day the same or are there days you particularly dislike?'

'Tuesdays and Thursdays,' Rajesh replied. 'They're the worst.'

'What happens on those days?'

Rajesh hadn't really thought about that before. He'd just instinctively known he'd especially not wanted to go to school on those days. 'We have assemblies then. We don't have them every day – the school's too big to have us all in together.'

'Do you feel the same in assembly as you do on buses and trains?'

Rajesh started to cry. 'What's wrong with me? I'm so frightened of everything – I hate going anywhere now. I want to stay home all the time.'

'I think you've developed a phobia, Rajesh. Perhaps even agoraphobia. Have you heard that word before?'

Rajesh nodded. 'But I'm not sure what it means.' He felt more confident about talking to the counsellor now. She seemed to understand, and that made him feel better. She hadn't laughed at him. He was glad he'd got some of his bad feelings off his chest.

The counsellor explained to Rajesh how lots of people feel frightened in crowds, needing to escape and be in a place where they feel safe. She offered to make him an appointment to see a psychologist, if he wanted. She'd write a note to his parents so that they could discuss the idea and give him time to think about it. Listening to her gave him time to calm down before he left the room. He felt a huge relief. He wasn't going mad, he had a definite problem that someone could help him with.

Discussion Sheet 8: It Happened One Day

1. Has anything ever happened to you to make you dread a repeat of the situation? If so, how did you feel and what did you do about it?

2. What is a phobia?

3. List any phobias you have. (Most people have at least one.)

4. How do you deal with these phobias?

5. (a) Do you, or does someone you know, have a phobia that interferes with everyday life?

   (b) What phobias do you know of?

6. (a) Rajesh was suffering from panic attacks. What are they?

   (b) Can you describe how he might have felt during a panic attack and the reaction his body has to the panic?

7. Very often, people who suffer from panic attacks and general phobias such as agoraphobia (specific phobias include fear of spiders, heights, snakes, birds…) hide their problems because they are worried about being made fun

of. How would you react to someone confiding in you about a phobia?

8. (a) Are phobias something to be ashamed of?

    (b) Are some phobias more socially acceptable than others? If so, why?

9. How far would you allow a phobia to affect your life before seeking help? Or would you take great pains to hide it, whatever the cost?

10. Rajesh found it difficult to start talking about his feelings. How did the school counsellor encourage him to talk?

Leader Sheet 8: It Happened One Day

1. **Has anything ever happened to you to make you dread a repeat of the situation? If so, how did you feel and what did you do about it?**
   (Personal responses required.)

2. **What is a phobia?**
   A phobia is a great, irrational fear of, and wish to avoid, a particular object or situation. Many people have minor phobias that may cause them some distress but do not stop them from leading normal, everyday lives. When the fear greatly disturbs a person and interferes with his or her life, as in Rajesh's case, they need professional help.

3. **List any phobias you have. (Most people have at least one.)**
   (Personal response required.)

4. **How do you deal with these phobias?**
   (Personal response required.)

5. **(a) Do you, or does someone you know, have a phobia that interferes with everyday life?**
   (Personal response required.)

   (b) What phobias do you know of?

Phobia		Fear
Acrophobia	⇨	Fear of heights
Aerophobia	⇨	Fear of flying
Anemophobia	⇨	Fear of wind
Apipophobia	⇨	Fear of bees
Arachnophobia	⇨	Fear of spiders
Brontophobia	⇨	Fear of storms
Claustrophobia	⇨	Fear of enclosed spaces
Cynophobia	⇨	Fear of dogs
Emetophobia	⇨	Fear of vomiting
Erythrophobia	⇨	Fear of blushing
Gatophobia	⇨	Fear of cats
Helminthophobia	⇨	Fear of worms
Haematophobia	⇨	Fear of blood
Hodophobia	⇨	Fear of travel
Kakorraphiaphobia	⇨	Fear of failure

Katagelophobia	⇨	*Fear of ridicule*
Maieusiophobia	⇨	*Fear of pregnancy*
Maniophobia	⇨	*Fear of insanity*
Musophobia	⇨	*Fear of mice*
Mysophobia	⇨	*Fear of dirt*
Necrophobia	⇨	*Fear of death*
Ochlophobia	⇨	*Fear of crowds*
Odontophobia	⇨	*Fear of dental work*
Ophiophobia	⇨	*Fear of snakes*
Ornithophobia	⇨	*Fear of birds*
Pnigerophobia	⇨	*Fear of smothering*
Scholionophobia	⇨	*Fear of school*
Triskaedekaphobia	⇨	*Fear of the number thirteen*
Trypanophobia	⇨	*Fear of injections*
Zoophobia	⇨	*Fear of animals*

6. (a) *Rajesh was suffering from panic attacks. What are they?*

A panic attack is an unreasonably large response to a small event. People get panic attacks when they have non-specific fears in a situation where they feel ill at ease or remember an unpleasant event. (Unlike the reaction of a person who has a fear of spiders – their fear is centred on the spider, but once the spider has been removed, they are OK.)

A person's first panic attack is usually because of something physical, such as feeling ill on a bus, and the person worries about public humiliation. Then the person fears it may happen again and starts to fear the fear, not the original cause. It is the person's fear that produces all the unpleasant symptoms.

It is then very easy for this fear to spiral out of control, so that the person suffers panic attacks for a great number of reasons in a number of situations. The person usually either needs to escape, or may faint or vomit.

(b) *Can you describe how he might have felt during a panic attack and the reaction his body has to the panic?*

How Rajesh might feel:

* Ashamed of his reactions.

* Confused, not knowing what was happening to him.

* Faint.

* Isolated and miserable.

- Nauseous.
- Not knowing where to turn.
- Terrified.
- Wanting to escape.
- Weak.

How Rajesh's body might react:

- Being sick.
- Chest pains.
- Difficulty swallowing.
- Dry mouth.
- Fainting.
- Muscle pains.
- Needing to open his bowels.
- Needing to urinate.
- Rapid heart rate.
- Ringing in the ears.
- Shaking.
- Sweating.

7. *Very often, people who suffer from panic attacks and general phobias such as agoraphobia (specific phobias include fear of spiders, heights, snakes, birds...) hide their problems because they are worried about being made fun of. How would you react to someone confiding in you about a phobia?*

- Seriously (a friend's problem is not to be made fun of).
- Sympathetically (you might try to comfort your friend as well as listening in a caring way).
- With understanding (if not of the problem itself then of the distress it is causing).
- Practically (suggest where to go for help and offer to go with the person).

8. **(a) Are phobias something to be ashamed of?**

Having a phobia can ruin someone's life. The person should not be made to feel ashamed of it but often does – probably because when in a panic, he or she loses control, and people are not very understanding of mental health problems.

(b) Are some phobias more socially acceptable than others? If so why?

Some phobias *are* more socially acceptable. Generally, people are quite happy to talk about their fear of spiders, heights, snakes and mice. These are very common phobias and do not tend to interfere with everyday lives. But not so with agoraphobia, where people fear leaving the house, going into shops or travelling on public transport. For non-sufferers, this is hard to understand, so they find it hard to be sympathetic. They can see no real danger in travelling on a bus, for example, whereas they can with snakes or heights.

9. **How far would you allow a phobia to affect your life before seeking help? Or would you take great pains to hide it, whatever the cost?**

(Personal response required.)

10. **Rajesh found it difficult to start talking about his feelings. How did the school counsellor encourage him to talk?**

   - By not rushing him.
   - By gently prompting him.
   - By letting him explain in his own good time and in his own way.
   - By being non-judgemental. (She didn't say, 'That's a bit silly, now.')
   - By not being shocked or surprised by what she heard.
   - By accepting what he said and accepting the level of his distress. She didn't belittle his experiences. (She didn't say things like, 'Don't you think that's a bit of an exaggeration?')
   - By being sympathetic.
   - By being understanding. (She'd heard it all before and knew about what he was going through.)

STORY 9: *Preeti's Lost Bracelet*

A splash of yellow showed underneath Preeti's cuff. 'What's that?' asked Sally.

'My uncle bought it for me,' Preeti said, showing off her wrist.

'Let me see,' Malika asked. Soon a group of girls had gathered around Preeti, admiring her new bracelet. Preeti had a lot of gold jewellery.

Preeti's mother had told her not to wear the bracelet yet, as it was a bit too big for her. She had tiny, delicate wrists and although the bracelet was small, she did need to grow a little more before it would fit her properly.

That afternoon, Preeti's class had games and they played rounders on the field. Back in the changing rooms, Preeti found she had lost her bracelet!

'Why didn't you hand in your bracelet, Preeti, when I collected all the valuables?' asked Miss Flaherty, the games teacher.

Preeti shrugged her shoulders miserably. She had liked it so much she hadn't wanted to part with it, even for a double lesson.

'We don't have time to look for it now – you'll have to search after school,' Miss Flaherty told her.

At the end of the day, Preeti's bracelet was still missing, even though her friends had helped look for it. What would her uncle say if she didn't find it by the next time he visited? And what would her mum say?

Two weeks later, Sally and Malika took a short cut across the field on their way home. As they stepped off the path onto the grass, Sally saw something glisten. It was lying in the crevice between the path and the field, hidden by weeds. Sally stooped down and quickly fished out the bracelet to put in her pocket.

'What was that?' Malika asked curiously.

'What was what?' Sally replied innocently.

'I saw you put something in your pocket.' Malika stopped walking, waiting for an answer.

'Oh, I dropped my hanky,' Sally muttered.

'Let me see,' Malika demanded.

'Malika!' Sally uttered in disgust, pretending to think Malika sick for wanting to examine a snotty hanky.

'Hankies don't jingle,' Malika pointed out. Sally blushed. She had been caught out. 'Let me see.' Malika held out her hand expectantly.

Reluctantly, Sally showed her. 'I found it. It's mine,' she defended.

'But it's Preeti's! You can't keep it. It doesn't belong to you.'

'But Preeti didn't look after it. She's got loads of other things. She won't miss it,' Sally told Malika stubbornly.

'You know how upset Preeti's been. You must give it back. It's stealing if you don't.'

'Not if you find something. If you found a five-pound note in the street, would you hand it in to the police?' Sally challenged.

'I don't know,' Malika admitted. 'But if I saw the person drop it I would definitely give it back. What would you do with the bracelet anyway? You couldn't ever wear it.'

Sally had acted instinctively and hadn't considered what she'd do with the bracelet or the guilt she would feel every time she saw Preeti. Malika was right, it was stealing and she felt dreadfully ashamed. Sally handed over the bracelet. 'You won't ever tell her I wanted to keep it, will you?'

Malika considered. 'I think you've learned your lesson. But if anything else goes missing in future you will be the first person I think of, whether you stole it or not.'

Discussion Sheet 9: Preeti's Lost Bracelet

1. Should Preeti have worn her bracelet to school?

2. Did Preeti deserve to lose her bracelet, as she did not hand it in to Miss Flaherty?

3. Why did Sally put the bracelet in her pocket when she found it?

4. 'Finders keepers, losers weepers.' Do you believe in this rhyme?

5. If you had been Sally and had found the bracelet when Malika was not there to stop you, would you have kept it?

6. If you were Preeti and found out what Sally had tried to do, how would you react?

7. (a) If you found someone's diary, would you read it and use the entries to make fun of the person or would you hand it back unread?

    (b) Is something personal, like a diary, as important as something valuable?

8. How would you feel if someone found your diary and read it?

9. (a) Was Malika right to tell Sally to return the bracelet?

    (b) Are you very definite in your views on what is right and what is wrong? Or do you feel at times there is no clear dividing line?

10. (a) Was it fair of Malika to brand Sally a thief for as long as she would know her?

    (b) Would you have felt the same way if you were Malika?

    (c) How would it feel to be Sally?

Leader Sheet 9: Preeti's Lost Bracelet

1. **Should Preeti have worn her bracelet to school?**

    No valuable jewellery should be worn to school – it's a temptation to others to steal it and a big responsibility to look after it. Also, her mum had told her not to wear it.

2. **Did Preeti deserve to lose her bracelet, as she did not hand it in to Miss Flaherty?**

    No, she didn't. She just hadn't been sensible and if she'd thought about it, she'd have known there was a good chance of losing it, as it didn't even fit her.

3. **Why did Sally put the bracelet in her pocket when she found it?**

    She had coveted the bracelet. She'd seen it and wanted it for herself and was jealous that her friend had so many nice pieces of jewellery.

4. **'Finders keepers, losers weepers.' Do you believe in this rhyme?**

    Yes:

    - If it's a small amount of money that belongs to a stranger, whom you can't identify. (If you felt guilty about keeping it you could give it to charity.)

    No:

    - Not if you know to whom the property belongs.
    - Not if the person will suffer from the loss of whatever you find. It might be a great deal of money or it might be a valuable piece of jewellery that has sentimental value and can never be replaced.

5. **If you had been Sally and had found the bracelet when Malika was not there to stop you, would you have kept it?**

    (Personal response required.)

6. **If you were Preeti and found out what Sally had tried to do, how would you react?**

    You might be hurt, feeling it wasn't a friendly thing to do, especially since she knew how upset you'd been. You might be very angry with her and want nothing more to do with her, feeling she'd betrayed your trust.

7. **(a) If you found someone's diary, would you read it and use the entries to make fun of the person or would you hand it back unread?**

(Personal response required.)

(b) Is something personal, like a diary, as important as something valuable?

Possibly, depending on how revealing the entries were. Once a stolen piece of jewellery is given back, it's back with you. But when a diary has been read, the intimacy is lost and the private information can be shared with others even after the diary has been returned.

8. **How would you feel if someone found your diary and read it?**
   - That the person had stolen a part of you.
   - That your entries in the diary had been cheapened.
   - That your privacy had been invaded.
   - Violated.

9. **(a) Was Malika right to tell Sally she had to return the bracelet?**
   Yes. If she didn't make Sally return the bracelet, she too would have been responsible for Preeti's loss. And Preeti was friends with both of them. Imagine how she would feel if she found out the two of them had conspired against her.

   (b) Are you very definite in your views on what is right and what is wrong? Or do you feel at times there is no clear dividing line?
   (Personal response required.)

   (Sometimes there's no clear dividing line – you have to go by your gut instincts and do what feels right at the time.)

10. **(a) Was it fair of Malika to brand Sally a thief for as long as she would know her?**
    No: It wasn't fair, but Malika was so angry on her friend's behalf that she wanted to hurt Sally as much as possible. It would have been kinder if Malika had kept those thoughts to herself, but at least Sally

knew where she stood. Malika was very blunt with her but it might stop her from doing something silly in the future.

Yes: It was fair because stealing is wrong and it was even more wrong to steal from a friend. The bracelet was a personal gift from Preeti's uncle, not an anonymous or replaceable five-pound note, for example.

(b) Would you have felt the same way if you were Malika?

(Personal response required.)

(c) How would it feel to be Sally?

Sally probably wished she could rewind the clock and point out the bracelet to Malika straight away. She would feel ashamed and guilty about what she'd done.

STORY 10: *Just One Last Game*

Mrs Hirani saw her son was still playing with his computer. 'Sanjay, have you done your homework yet?'

'Not yet. I'm just about to start.' Sanjay didn't take his eyes off the monitor.

'Now, Sanjay! It's getting late and you'll be too tired for school.' Sanjay just kept pressing the buttons on the joystick. His mother went downstairs. 'Aran, he's *still* playing and hasn't done his homework again. We only see him at mealtimes – and when we do see him, he's miles away. He never listens to a word we say. I wish we'd never bought him that computer.'

Aran sighed. His son was entitled to enjoy himself but it wasn't healthy to sit for hours in front of a computer.

Sanjay finished his game, but was disappointed with his score. His history essay would have to wait. Just one last game...

Aran came into Sanjay's room very softly. He wanted to see for himself what effect these games were having on his son. It was after 9pm and Sanjay still hadn't opened his school bag. Aran felt angry. This wasn't why they had made sacrifices and worked hard to provide for Sanjay. He bent down to switch off the electrical socket.

'Dad! I was nearly there! It was going to be my best score yet!' Sanjay protested.

'The only score I'm interested in is what you get for your school work. You told me your friends had computers to help them with school. As far as I know you haven't used a single educational programme I bought for you and you haven't used it to type out your essays! Now get your homework done. And I don't want to see you playing games for longer than half an hour each day!' Aran watched his son take out his books. Once satisfied that Sanjay had finally got down to work he left to go back downstairs.

Sanjay found the essay hard. He couldn't concentrate as he was so annoyed about his dad messing up that last game. It would have meant he'd have beaten Mark and Richard. He knew it would...

He battled with his essay but it was too hard. Perhaps he'd be able to copy from someone at school, if he got in early. It didn't have to be handed in until breaktime. He looked longingly at the computer.

After 11pm, all was quiet and Sanjay put on his dressing gown and the light at his desk. He quietly lowered the switch on the wall socket and heard the computer hum into life. One last game…

Aran got up to go to the toilet and saw the faint beam of light from under Sanjay's door. He rushed in to catch the guilty look and the flashing screen. Putting an end to it once and for all, he grabbed the scissors that lay on the desk, unplugged the machine and cut the plug off the end.

'Tomorrow that computer's going in the loft!'

The day went badly for Sanjay. He couldn't find anyone to copy from. He'd asked too many times before. This was the third homework he'd missed that week and all the teachers had commented in his homework diary. His parents had to sign it at the end of the week.

Sanjay tried to catch up that evening but couldn't settle, finding it hard to sit still and to concentrate. He needed to have a game to get him in the mood to work. Although he knew that he wouldn't get his computer back from the loft until his schoolwork was back to the same standard he just couldn't do it. He just couldn't…

Discussion Sheet 10: Just One Last Game

1. (a) How had Sanjay become addicted to computer games?

    (b) How was it affecting his life?

2. Was Aran unfair to his son? Give reasons for your answer.

3. Why had the computer been bought in the first place?

4. Have your parents or guardians ever bought you something that they later regretted? If so, what was it and why did they regret it?

5. (a) People claim that playing computer games improves reaction times. What are they?

   (b) Do you think that achieving improved reaction times justifies the time spent playing these games?

6. Have you played with computer games? If so, what effect did it have? Can you understand how Sanjay felt?

7. What other things can give withdrawal symptoms when taken away? Try to give as many examples as you can.

8. Have you experienced some form of addiction other than to computer games?

9. What do you think are the warning signs that you are becoming addicted to something?

10. Why can addictions be dangerous?

Leader Sheet 10: Just One Last Game

1. (a) How had Sanjay become addicted to computer games?

He enjoyed playing the games but it had become important that he beat his friends' scores at any cost. He couldn't stop, hoping that the next score would always be better than the last – a bit like a gambler telling him or herself that next time they'll win, but they never, or rarely, do.

(b) How was it affecting his life?

- Sanjay did nothing else and thought of nothing else but the games.

- He was not doing his schoolwork and could not settle down to think about it.

- He was relying on copying from friends – but now they were refusing him, not liking him using them in this way.

- He was getting very behind and probably did not understand the work.

- It was affecting the relationship he had with his parents – his mother said they only saw him at mealtimes and even then he was distracted.

2. Was Aran unfair to his son? Give reasons for your answer.

No: He wasn't unfair, because Sanjay obviously could not stop even when his father had told him he must do his homework. His father had said that he could still play games each day but that they would be limited to half an hour, which was reasonable under the circumstances. Sanjay had switched the computer back on in secret. As he had no self-control over his playing, his father had to take over and ensure that Sanjay had no choice but to stop.

Yes: He was unfair, because he should have talked it over with Sanjay, recognising that his son had a problem and couldn't stop. Aran could try to 'wean' him off by providing other forms of entertainment. (However, this assumes that his father has sufficient insight to understand about addictions. It also doesn't take into account his father's anger and disappointment in his son, having used his hard-earned money to buy Sanjay something that should help with school, but finding it had done the opposite.)

3. ***Why had the computer been bought in the first place?***

So that Sanjay could type out his essays and learn from the educational disks. Sanjay's father had also bought it because his son had told him his friends had computers and he didn't want his son 'left behind'. He was keen for his son to do well at school.

4. ***Have your parents or guardians ever bought you something that they later regretted? If so, what was it and why did they regret it?***

(Personal responses required.)

5. ***(a) People claim that playing computer games improves reaction times. What are they?***

Reaction times are measures of how quickly you can respond to something that happens. The faster your reaction time, the more alert and responsive you are. When you are competing against your friends at computer games, much may depend on the speed of your reaction. However, in life, fast reaction times are not that important. When you drive, you do need to respond quickly, but few can maintain the level of alertness required to have a very fast response. That is why stopping distances have reaction times built in because it is well-known that cars continue to travel for a short time after the driver has seen the need to stop, before the brakes are applied.

(b) Do you think that achieving improved reaction times justifies the time spent playing these games?

No. Even if you played computer games regularly, there is a limit to how much your reaction time can be improved. We are often looking at a fraction of a second, which is a very small length of time. Considering that you cannot change the speed at which the brain signals a hand to move, practising will only produce a small improvement.

Note: Some games have caused epileptic fits in players, particularly those games that have vivid, flashing screens. It is safer to play them in a well-lit room so that there is little contrast between the brightness of the screen and the background lighting. You can also turn the contrast/brightness button down on the monitor. These precautions lessen the effect of the flashing lights. It is also advisable to take regular breaks – say twenty minutes every hour.

6. ***Have you played with computer games? If so, what effect did it have? Can you understand how Sanjay felt?***

(Personal responses required.)

7. ***What other things can give withdrawal symptoms when taken away? Try to give as many examples as you can.***

- Alcohol and tobacco (legal mood-altering drugs); narcotic drugs (illegal mood-altering drugs, such as heroin, opium, cocaine, LSD, ecstasy and cannabis); tranquillisers (prescription drugs, such as Valium); amphetamines (stimulants – can be prescribed or illegally obtained); caffeine in tea, coffee and soft drinks such as Coca Cola; and chocolate.

- Other addictions include gambling, running (or other sport activities), over-work (workaholics). With these addictions, the person becomes addicted to his or her own body's adrenaline and endorphins. The increased levels are missed when the activity is stopped. (Endorphins are produced within the body to reduce the perception of pain and are similar to opiates. Adrenaline, produced in flight or fight responses, is similar to amphetamines.)

- Gambling and compulsive shopping (when people buy things they do not really want or need) may also cause psychological changes that produce a need to continue the activity.

8. ***Have you experienced some form of addiction other than to computer games?***

When someone first starts having sex, or discovers the pleasure of masturbation, he or she may be able to think of nothing else and become 'addicted'. Also, many children are 'addicted' to television – they may not know how to amuse themselves without it and be grumpy if they can no longer watch it.

9. ***What do you think are the warning signs that you are becoming addicted to something?***

- Doing the 'thing' 'on the quiet' or in secret.

- Not being able to stop, even when you think you should or would like to.
- The 'thing' becoming more important than schoolwork – or paid work.
- Not bothering to eat sensibly or forgetting to eat altogether.
- Being irritable when you have a break from the 'thing'.
- Finding it hard to relax or sleep.
- Having big mood changes.
- Not caring about anything apart from the 'thing'.
- Losing friends because the 'thing' has become more important.
- Becoming harder to understand and get on with.

10. Why can addictions be dangerous?

Addictions can be dangerous because certain things in excess can harm the body. The person can become drug-dependent or totally dependent on the activity (such as drinking) for support and comfort. The person risks losing touch with reality and the addiction can take over his or her life. The person may no longer care about personal appearance or the standard of work he or she performs. Addictions can lead to loss of the person's job and family, friends and home.

STORY 11: A Better Class of People

Bharti Hirani was up first. She noticed the smell as soon as she was on the stairs to go down. It didn't take long to find the source, but what a mess! Most of it was on the mat but some had fallen onto her new carpet. Bharti quickly got to work, disposing of the doormat and scrubbing and disinfecting the carpet. There were no traces left when it was time for the rest of the family to come for breakfast.

'That's the girl from the Paki family that moved in next to Mrs Roberts,' Charlotte told her friend, Saffron. 'Dad says they're the first on our road and have lowered the tone of the neighbourhood. The house prices will probably fall now. He can't understand how they had the money to buy the house.'

Amita saw the two girls standing chatting at the corner of her road. They looked about her age but she knew from their uniform that they didn't go to her school. She hoped they could be friends, as she didn't know anyone close by.

As Amita approached the girls, they turned to face her fully, barring her path. If Amita were to pass, she'd have to go onto the road.

'Where do you think you're going?' Charlotte demanded.

'Home,' Amita said timidly.

'A bit far from the airport aren't you?' Saffron asked.

Amita tried to pass but Charlotte blocked her movement. 'What sort of uniform's that?' Charlotte flicked Amita's tie.

'Queensbury High. Can I go now?' Amita now knew they would never be friends.

'I suppose your dad couldn't afford to change schools as well as house,' Saffron sneered.

'There was no need. I'm happy where I am. It's a good school,' Amita murmured. Amita shuddered at the thought of going to their private school. A waste of money if that's how they were taught to behave.

Saffron pushed Amita. 'You're nobody. Nobody, do you understand? You don't belong here. You're the wrong colour for a start.'

Amita was stunned. She hadn't realised this was purely racial – she had plenty of white friends at school.

'I bet you've got three families living in that house of yours to help pay for it,' Charlotte declared.

Amita frowned. 'No. My father's a doctor. It's a good job.'

'What sort of doctor? Witch doctor?' Charlotte laughed.

'Witch doctors are African,' Amita replied quietly.

'You must think you're so clever – but no one here wants you. We don't want Pakis on our street.' Charlotte pulled Amita's tie to emphasise her words before stepping aside to let her pass.

Mrs Hirani was puzzled over Amita's behaviour. They normally had a cup of tea together when she got in but now she kept going straight upstairs to do her homework. She sighed. The family had moved here because her husband had wanted his children to be brought up in a good 'professional' area. But she hated leaving the house now as people stared at her. These were what Nikhil had called 'a better class of people'.

The door banged and Ramesh came in. He had caught a later train than Amita. Bharti went into the hall to say hello but stopped in her tracks. Ramesh's shirt was torn, his tie was missing and he had been crying.

Bharti knew she now had to tell Nikhil about the dog turd that had been shoved through the letter box. It was no use pretending. A better class of people indeed!

Discussion Sheet 11: A Better Class of People

Please note that after the Second World War, Britain was only too glad to welcome Africans and Asians to do the work the British disliked and to increase manpower following the deaths of the British soldiers.

1. (a) What is racism?

    (b) How would you describe racist people?

2. (a) Which are acceptable words, or expressions, to describe people from different cultures to yourself and which are abusive?

    (b) What makes a word abusive?

3. How do racism and the myths surrounding racist ideas get passed down generations?

4. (a) Why do people make racist remarks?

    (b) What do they gain from it?

5. (a) Can you think of comments that you have heard to put down blacks and Asians?

    (b) Can they be backed up by fact?

6. Does the colour of your skin or your place of birth make you a better person? Or, indeed, your parents' or guardians' bank balance?

7. What racial attacks take place other than those brought up in the story?

8. What effect do racist comments and racist attacks have on children from ethnic minority groups?

9. (a) Can you think of racist comments or myths spread between different groups of white people?

    (b) Can they be backed up by fact?

10. Is there anything the Hirani family could do to improve their situation? (Moving house again is not an option.)

Leader Sheet 11: A Better Class of People

---

1. (a) *What is racism?*

- Racism is the assumption that one's own race is superior to another.

- It is often accompanied by prejudice against members of different ethnic groups. (Prejudice is having a preconceived opinion over whether or not you like something. It is not based on fact.)

- Racism has been used to justify discrimination, verbal and physical abuse and even genocide (the deliberate killing of an entire race or ethnic group).

(b) *How would you describe racist people?*

- Biased – they favour particular racial groups at the expense of others.

- Dangerous – they can spread hatred and incite racial attacks.

- Ignorant – they make judgements without factual knowledge and believe in stereotypes (attributing certain negative traits to an entire cultural group).

- Intolerant – of anyone different to themselves.

- Narrow-minded – they can only see a limited view of the world around them.

- Opinionated – they are not willing to have their opinions changed but are happy to tell everyone about them, however wrong their opinions may be.

- Shallow – they won't look beyond the person's skin to recognise his or her personality or similarities to themselves. They concentrate on visible differences.

- Stubborn – they are fixed in their views and don't want to change their minds.

2. (a) *Which are acceptable words, or expressions, to describe people from different cultures to yourself and which are abusive?*

Note: Some words that are unacceptable to use today were considered the most appropriate many years back. For example, in the nineteenth century, 'black' and 'nigger' were used. Later, in the twentieth century, both these names were dropped and replaced by 'negro'. In the 1960s, 'nigger' and 'negro' were considered racist and 'black' was reinstated.

Acceptable words or expressions:

- Anti-Semitic instead of 'anti-Jewish'.
- Black (it is unacceptable to use this term for Indians, Pakistanis and Bangladeshis).
- Asian, Caucasian (referring to a white person), Chinese, African, African-Caribbean.
- Inuit.
- Indigenous American.
- Foreign national or non-national (not 'foreigner').
- Undocumented person or undocumented resident (not 'illegal immigrant' or 'illegal alien').

Unacceptable words or expressions:

Bagel-bender	Used to refer to a Jewish person – bagels are the bread rings that Jewish people traditionally eat.
Chink	This comes from a mispronunciation of the Chinese word for China, 'Chung-kuo'.
Coon	This may come from the last syllable of the Portuguese word for buildings put up to hold slaves before they were sold – 'barracoës' – or from the word raccoon (a black-faced rural pest). 'Egg and spoon' is the rhyming slang version of coon.
Dago	This is used to refer to someone of Hispanic (Spanish or Latin American) origin, derived from the name Diego (James). It is also used as an insult to people, usually male, of any Mediterranean origin.
Darkie	This is used to refer to a black or Asian person.
Dark meat	This is used when non-white people are referred to as sex objects.
Eskimo	This is no longer a politically correct term. Inuit is preferred. Those living in Alaska use the term 'native Alaskan'.
Gook	Used of East Asians in general. It is from Korea. Korea is 'han-kuk', America is 'mei-kuk'. (Kuk means person.) The term was used by US soldiers in the Vietnam war and earlier in a Filipino uprising (from the Filipino word, 'gugus').

Gringo	Used by Latin Americans of North Americans and Europeans. US soldiers were often heard singing, 'Green Grow the Lilacs' in Mexico in 1848. Locals joined the first two words together.
Gyp/gyppo	Used to refer to gypsies. (It was mistakenly thought that they originated from Egypt, hence the name, gypsy.)
Hookie	Used to refer to Jewish people (referring to 'hooked' noses).
Immigrant	Used to refer to non-white people who immigrated to Britain.
Itinerant	Used to refer to gypsies but can also be applied to non-gypsies who follow a travelling lifestyle.
Lick of the tarbrush	This is used to refer to people of black or sub-continental Indian origin.
Jew/Jewess	Use Jewish or Jewish person. (Saying 'He's a Jew' is now frowned upon. Say 'He is Jewish'.)
Jock	Nickname for Scottish men.
Jungle bunny	Used to refer to African-Caribbeans but also used by Australians when referring to Aborigines and South Sea Islanders.
Kraut	Used to refer to a German person (replacing 'Hun' and 'Jerry'). From the German word for pickled cabbage, 'sauerkraut'.
Ivan	Nickname for Russian men.
Negro	This has been dropped because it is too similar to the word 'nigger'. 'Negress' is an even bigger no-no.
Nigger	This is used to refer to a black person and is derived from the Latin for black, 'niger', via Spanish ('negro') and French ('ngère').
Nig-nog	This is used to refer to a black person and is derived from nigger.
Nip	Used to refer to Japanese (from the word 'Nippon', Japanese for Japan).
Non-white	There is a feeling of superiority of white here: there are whites and the non-whites (all lumped together in one insignificant bundle).
Paddy	Used to refer to Irishmen (from the name Patrick).
Paki	Used loosely to refer to Pakistanis and Indian sub-continentals.
Red Indian	This and 'Redskin' are considered racist. The colour red was dropped first and the people were called

	'American Indians'. Then any reference to the word 'Indian' became no longer politically correct because the word Indian is associated with the Indian sub-continent (the name 'Indian' was used by mistake in the fifteenth century – someone got their geography wrong) and because in the cowboy and Indian films, it is always the 'Indians' that are the 'baddies'. Now they are called 'indigenous Americans'. (Also, sometimes, 'native Americans', although this is not wholly acceptable because it also refers to the first settlers.)
Sambo	Used to refer to a black person, usually male. It dates back to the slave trade in America.
Spade	This refers to black people and is from the expression 'as black as the ace of spades'. (It has nothing to do with the expression, 'to call a spade a spade' – this phrase is from the Ancient Greeks referring to someone who speaks very openly.)
Spick/spic	This refers to people of Italian or Hispanic origin, making fun of the way they speak. ('No spik English.')
Spook	Used in America to refer to black people, either from the idea of black spectres or because of their 'haunting' certain locations.
Taffy	Used to refer to Welshmen (from the Welsh name Dafydd, pronounced 'Davvith' [David]).
Wog	Used to refer to dark-skinned people. The term is derived from some of the initials of 'Westernised Wily Oriental Gentleman' when referring to people working for the colonial British authorities. Another possible origin is from the word 'golliwog' – a black doll with curly hair.
Wop	From the word 'guappo' meaning robust. It was the name given to Italian youths who migrated to America.
Yank	This refers to Americans or people who live in the USA. It was first used in the form of Yankee and is connected with the early Dutch settlers.
Yid	This is Yiddish (a Germanic dialect influenced by Hebrew) for a Yiddish-speaking Jewish person, but is used in English as a derogatory term against all Jewish people.
Zulu	This is used as a term of abuse for black people by British people.

(b) What makes a word abusive?

A word is made abusive by the way it is said (such as with derision) and by the way it is used – to imply that one race is superior to another or to make fun of another race, using terms with disrespect. For example, many of the above are not 'proper' names but cruel nicknames designed to hurt and demean.

3. **How do racism and the myths surrounding racist ideas get passed down generations?**

When people are racially prejudiced, they often stereotype (hold fixed or exaggerated perceptions about a race or ethnic group). They may be exaggerating something they have heard, or basing their opinion of an entire race on one incident known to them about one member of that race. (For example, the opinion that 'black people cause trouble' may have been held in a family because of something one black person did and is then applied to the entire race. However, a white person would not dream of applying the same thought process to a member of his or her own race from one incident alone.)

Stereotypes become fixed in people's minds so that, over a period of time, they become thought of as factual despite there being evidence to the contrary.

Racial jokes are also responsible for myths about racist ideas being spread and held as true.

Racist ideas are also perpetuated by children. They look up to their parents or guardians who, early on in their lives, are the only source of information. They listen and respect their views and hold their views as true (children can repeat their parents' or guardians' expressions verbatim) and accept them without question. It is then harder to change the child's point of view even when he or she is older. Even if this does happen, the child may have to hide his or her enlightenment from parents or guardians who are so racist they will not tolerate any other viewpoint.

Note: Often people are racist within their own culture – it is not just a problem between whites and blacks or Asians. Within Indian society, for example, there are many castes and there is prejudice between one caste and another, and a feeling of superiority among members of a high caste.

4. **(a) Why do people make racist remarks?**

It is a form of bullying and makes the person feel superior.

(b) What do they gain from it?

It can lead to discrimination (despite this being illegal) where the preferred races are given preferential treatment such as in job applications and wages.

5. **(a) Can you think of comments that you have heard to put down blacks and Asians?**

- In the story, it was mentioned that Amita probably shared her home with other families to help pay for it. There are two issues here. One is that Asians don't mind 'slumming' and squeezing in as many bodies into a home as possible, and the other is the assumption that Asians can't have good jobs with high wages.

- 'There's no point in educating those Asian girls because they're married off young.' This implies that Asian women should not have a right to be educated and that they don't know what to do with their education when they do have it. It is also an oblique reference to arranged marriages. Do you have sufficient knowledge to make judgements here? Can you make judgements about cultures you don't thoroughly know and understand? Is your culture without fault? (Whichever culture it may be.)

- 'Blacks are trouble-makers.' How many do you know that are? How many do you know that aren't? Does it apply to all blacks? – Africans, African-Caribbean, second-generation 'British' blacks? American blacks? One cannot make such generalisations.

(b) Can they be backed up by fact?

No. Individual experiences may not be accurately applied to an entire race. (In a climate of racial tension, those on the receiving end of hatred and assaults may well behave negatively towards the group carrying out the racial attacks. This may confirm the attackers' views that their actions are justified for all of that culture.)

6. *Does the colour of your skin or your place of birth make you a better person? Or, indeed, your parents' or guardians' bank balance?*

No. What matters is:

- what you do
- who you become
- whether you have achieved your potential by doing your best
- how you live your life
- how you treat other people.

7. *What racial attacks take place other than those brought up in the story?*

People might:

- throw paint at the house
- put burning paper through the letter box
- graffitti the house
- threaten with, or use, a knife on another person
- mug the person, stealing his or her money
- spread untrue rumours about the person
- jeer at the person and encourage others to join in
- physically attack or kill the person.

8. *What effect do racist comments and racist attacks have on children from ethnic minority groups?*

- It makes them feel small and scared.
- They can underperform in school because of the stress and the constant barrage of demeaning comments about them (no one can thrive in an environment where they feel threatened and are abused).
- If the racial bullying is not effectively stopped, the child may be murdered, as Ahmed Ullah was in 1986. He was murdered in the schoolyard of Burnage School in Manchester by a white pupil.

- Living in fear, the child may become so disturbed that he or she commits suicide, as Vijay Singh, who was racially bullied, did in Manchester in 1996.

9. (a) Can you think of racist comments or myths spread between different groups of white people?

(Personal response required.)

(Think of racist remarks that might be made about the Irish, Welsh, Scottish, Americans, French, Italians, Jewish people.)

(b) Can they be backed up by fact?

No. There will always be some people within that culture that fulfil the myths – as in any culture. Unless you have irrefutable statistics to hand, avoid making any judgemental comments about any race or culture.

10. Is there anything the Hirani family could do to improve their situation? (Moving house again is not an option.)

- Ring up the heads of the bullies' school and ask them to help.
- Inform the police – racial attacks, abuse and threats are against the law.
- Speak to the parents of the children who had bullied theirs. (This is not always advisable – the parents may be proud of their children's behaviour and be part of the problem.)
- Try getting to know their neighbours so that any myths are dispelled. (They could, for example, throw a party and invite their neighbours; or chat to whoever they see in their garden as they walk past. This may not change things with the bullies as they may not be neighbours, but it would help to get the family accepted into the new community.)

STORY 12: *Slag!*

Anand was deep in thought, as he was most days. It didn't matter where he was or what he was supposed to be doing, he could not get his parents out of his mind.

They had separated about six months ago and had flaming rows, sometimes about who was going to have custody of him. Anand hated feeling he was the object of their hatred and his parents often used him to get back at each other. There was too much hurt all round and Anand felt he would explode with the frustration and unfairness of it all.

Last night was one of the worst. His dad had come round trying to make things less nasty but his mum wouldn't give a millimetre. She could not forgive him for being unfaithful and wanted nothing more to do with him.

Every time Dad asked her a question she would reply by saying to Anand, 'Tell your father…' She refused to talk directly to his dad even though they were in the same room. They seemed to have forgotten that he had any feelings at all. And to make it even worse, his mum was in such a foul mood by the time his dad left that she snapped at him until bedtime. Then he heard her crying over the telephone to Ravin, her boyfriend, who was the teacher at her evening class. Now that they were close, he often stayed overnight and Anand had to call him uncle.

Anand could understand his dad had done wrong, but could not understand why they couldn't sort it out. Once mum started seeing Ravin it was like half his dreams had been dashed because he'd always hoped – and still did – that they'd make it up. And then he could pretend that this nightmare had never happened.

Suddenly, he came to the present. The whole class had gone silent and was staring at him, including Miss Atkinson. He'd obviously been asked a question. 'Sorry…?'

Miss Atkinson for some unknown reason switched the question to someone else and the class relaxed into disappointment. They'd expected Anand to suffer the sharp end of her tongue. Anand sighed in relief.

Tracy giggled behind him. Her mum knew his mum and he always dreaded being near her. He ignored her.

'Your mum's a slag,' Tracy whispered, and she and her friend carried on giggling.

Anand felt all the pent-up hurt and frustration build into rage and boil over, and knew he'd lost control. He stood and picked up his stool, holding it above his head. Just before it left his hands, aimed at Tracy, Miss Atkinson roared, 'No!' and ran over. He stood still as she removed the stool.

'What's going on?' she asked sternly.

'She called my mum a slag.' Anand's voice was filled with indignation.

Tracy sat looking mutinous.

'It sounds as though you are too lippy for your own good, Tracy.' The class laughed. 'I want to see you both at break and we'll discuss it further.' She looked at Anand who was crying. 'Go and wait in the prep room. The technician will be there.' Then she continued with her lesson.

At break, Miss Atkinson saw Tracy first and told her how unkind she'd been. Then she saw Anand in private. 'Why did you react so violently, Anand?' she asked, crouching down to his level.

At first he was silent, but his teacher waited patiently.

'My mum's not a slag. Tracy keeps saying things about my parents that aren't true.'

'Have you got problems at home?'

Anand nodded, at first too choked to speak. 'My parents have split up and my mum's got a boyfriend.'

'You need to talk to someone. Bottling everything up is doing you no good. Would you like me to tell your Head of Year or your form teacher?'

'No.' His reply was strangled but firm.

'Have you told your parents how you feel?'

Anand shook his head.

'Then you must. They can't help you or make it easier if they don't know there's anything wrong. Will you promise me that you'll talk to them? You are too important not to.'

Anand nodded, feeling that she was right. It would be hard, but he'd do it. He wasn't going to be used as a weapon again.

Discussion Sheet 12: Slag!

1. (a) List Anand's problems. What effect are they having on his everyday life?

   (b) What emotions do you think children experience when their parents split up?

2. Do you agree with Miss Atkinson's advice? Why?

3. How would you stop your parents from using you as a weapon?

4. Should parents try to cover up the tension that exists between them? Why?

5. (a) Is it better for both parents to explain to their children that they have got problems?

   (b) Should children be told the reasons why?

6. Do you think parents should try to keep their marriage together at all costs for the sake of the children, or would there be less damage if they tried to have an amicable separation?

7. Is it the quality of upbringing that counts or the presence of both parents? Give reasons.

8. Can relationships with an absent parent improve? Is it likely that this parent will now make more effort with his or her children?

9. Do you see the remarriage of parents to new partners as a positive or negative thing? Why?

10. What messages do you think you might get about relationships if you experience the separation or divorce of your parents?

Leader Sheet 12: Slag!

1. **(a) List Anand's problems. What effect are they having on his everyday life?**

- He can't concentrate – it is affecting his schoolwork.

- He is completely absorbed in his problems at home – he allows himself no escape from his torments and is shutting himself off from other people.

- He feels powerless to change things – it makes him depressed and stressed.

- He doesn't like having to call his mum's boyfriend 'uncle' – it adds to his stress.

- He is very hurt – he will be afraid of getting hurt again and he may build an emotional wall around himself.

- He is unable to talk to anyone about his problems and his parents are too caught up in their problems to notice he needs help – he feels isolated.

- He is extremely sensitive about his parents – he reacted violently to Tracy's taunting.

The stress Anand is experiencing may harm his physical and mental health. He is certainly not enjoying life at the moment.

(b) What emotions do you think children experience when their parents split up?

- Anger – because of parents being unable to sort out their differences to avoid separation.

- Betrayal – they feel they have been let down in a major way.

- Blame – they may see their parents as being selfish and uncaring.

- Disbelief – up till then their parents have been one solid part of their lives that could be depended on not to change. Children believe their parents will always be there for them.

- Guilt – they mistakenly believe they are in some way to blame for what has happened and need to be reassured that this is not so.

- Insecurity and fear – as the unknown, unpredictable future looms ahead they are forced to adapt to a new lifestyle and maybe new people.
- Suspicion – they might find it harder to trust people and, if they can't trust their parents always to be there, who can they trust?

2. Do you agree with Miss Atkinson's advice? Why?

Yes: Anand must try to communicate with his parents and try to make things better. Someone has to explain to them what they are doing to him and he must protect himself from as much pain as possible. If he allowed the school to become involved, a teacher could act as intermediary between him and his parents. This would make his parents take what he has to say more seriously. If he could confide in his friends, they might be able to support him too.

No: His parents probably won't take any notice of him. (The pessimist's view – but there's nothing lost in trying.)

3. How would you stop your parents from using you as a weapon?

- By refusing to 'play' the game. Anand could have walked out when his mother asked him to be the go-between.
- By saying you can't stand them fighting and want to be left out of their arguments.
- By refusing to take sides.
- By telling another family member, such as a grandparent, about what is going on.

4. Should parents try to cover up the tension that exists between them? Why?

Yes:

- A child should not be brought into every small squabble so that he or she is constantly on edge. It is probably only once a major decision has been made that the child should be informed.

No:

- If the tension between parents is not possible to hide, yet they continue to deny to their questioning child that anything is wrong, the child is unlikely to be convinced, possibly causing more distress and mistrust in the long term.

- Trying to cover up gigantic tensions would put too great a strain on the parents – even if it were possible. It's better to explain what's going on rather than leave it to the child's frightened imagination.

5. (a) Is it better for both parents to explain to their children that they have got problems?

Yes. Then the child doesn't get a different version from each parent, and that is likely to be more reassuring.

(b) Should the children be told the reasons why?

- Once a couple have decided to separate, they should have frank and open conversations with their children about what will happen in the future.
- The child could perhaps better understand that it's not his or her fault. When no reasons are given for the problems, the child may blame him or herself.

6. Do you think parents should try to keep their marriage together at all costs for the sake of the children, or would there be less damage if they tried to have an amicable separation?

Living unhappily for years takes its toll on all family members. Unless you can live quite amicably on the surface for a long time, it may be less damaging to admit to the children that there are problems and explain what you are going to do about them. Divorce may, for example, protect a child from an abusive parent.

7. Is it the quality of upbringing that counts or the presence of both parents? Give reasons.

There is no easy answer.

- The quality counts, but many children may be happy to sacrifice a bit of 'quality' to have a complete family with both parents providing care and acting as role models.
- If one parent is violent or has drug- or alcohol-related problems, the presence of that person in the family home may be more harmful to the happiness of the child.

- If parents are fighting most of the time, the quality of the upbringing may well be improved by having only one of them around.
- Both parents should not be present if the emotional cost of their being within the family group is too high, despite the presence of both parents being ideal (they complement one another and give balance to the family).
- There has been some debate on whether single mums can effectively discipline sons and some blame has been cast on absent fathers for their sons' anti-social and criminal behaviour.
- It is good for sons and daughters to have positive role models. If one parent is missing then the child of the same sex can lose out. (Assuming the parents do provide positive role models and assuming the parents are not a homosexual couple.)
- Every situation would have to be judged differently by the individuals involved.

8. Can relationships with an absent parent improve? Is it likely that this parent will now make more effort with his or her children?

- It is possible that once the strain of close family life is removed, the absent parent may get on better with his or her children and spouse.
- Guilt may prompt the absent parent to make a more concentrated effort during the short periods he or she may be caring for his or her children.
- It may depend on the reasons for the break-up. If there is anger and bitterness over what caused it, the presence of his or her unforgiving children may not help. If drugs or alcoholism or violence is involved, the break-up is further complicated.

9. Do you see the remarriage of parents to new partners as a positive or negative thing? Why?

Positive:

- Life may be calmer and may have settled down.
- Having additional people to care for you and consult may be good.

- You may enjoy being part of a larger family if the stepparents have children of their own that you get on with.

Negative:

- It may have made it definite that your own parents are never going to get back together.
- You may miss the absent parent terribly.
- You may view the stepparents as intruders in your home and in your other parent's home.
- You may not get on at all with your new family.

10. *What messages do you think you might get about relationships if you experience the separation or divorce of your parents?*

- You might feel that you shouldn't trust other people.
- You might think it risky to divulge your feelings in case you get hurt.
- You may have trouble expressing how you feel as you have experienced lack of communication between your parents and between you and your parents. These problems may extend to how you deal with your future partner.
- You might label all of the same sex as your 'bad' parent in the same way and so treat them without respect or fail to recognise that they have feelings.
- You might think that if a relationship is causing trouble you should walk out instead of trying to put it to rights. (You may not recognise that all marriages have their ups and downs. Statistics show that children of divorced parents are more likely to divorce themselves because the 'shame' of divorce is removed – their parents did it – and because they don't consider marriage worth fighting for.)

Section 2

Introduction

Section 2 is concerned with issues relevant to 12- to 15-year-olds. Stories 13 and 14 are interconnected with a bullying theme, although each story is complete in itself, and should be read in order. The rest of the stories in Section 2 can be read in any order. Some of the characters in this section also appear in later sections.

Story 24: I'm a Person Too can be read aloud as two parts: mother and daughter.

Summary of Contents

Story	Title	Subject
13	We Were Only Playing*	Bullying, in school
14	Chicken!*	Playing 'chicken', bullying
15	Honesty Policy	Tact versus honesty
16	Painful Puberty	Puberty changes and feelings
17	Nightmare	Video-nasties
18	I Fell Down the Stairs	Child abuse
19	I Don't Remember	Alcohol abuse
20	Joyrider	Joyriding, stealing cars
21	I Never Have Any Nice Clothes	Designer clothes, bullying
22	Shoplifter	Shoplifting, kleptomania
23	My Mum's Not Well	Obsessive–compulsive disorder
24	I'm a Person Too	Teenage and parental rights

* Titles in succession are interconnected and should be read in order.

STORY 13: We Were Only Playing

David Williams was squat, fat and wore glasses. He was very clever and such a goody-goody that Mark, Richard and Simon couldn't stand him.

'Give that back!' David cried as Richard grabbed his school bag.

'If you want it come and get it!' Richard taunted, holding out the bag at arm's length. As David lunged for it, Richard threw the bag to Mark. They laughed. David chased after it, pushing away the chairs that got in his way. His new calculator was in there – his dad would kill him if that got broken.

'Oh, look,' said Mark. 'Your bag wants to go out.' He pushed open the window from the second-floor classroom and let it hang for a tantalising moment so that David could watch it fall.

Just then the bell went and the three of them raced out to their next lesson, leaving David to pant after them to retrieve his bag. But when he got outside it was no longer there. And back at his lesson, he was told to stay behind after school for being late and not having the right equipment. He opened his mouth to protest but knew things would get worse if he grassed.

'Where's your bag?' Mrs Williams asked David as soon as he got home.

'I lost it.'

'Just like you lost your trainers and gym shorts?' David hung his head. 'Did you report it missing?'

'No.'

'No? How on earth can you lose things anyway? I want some straight answers and it had better be good or I don't know what your father will do. This has gone on long enough and I want to know the truth. Now!'

David told her of the weeks of torment and said he wasn't going back to school again. He couldn't stand it.

'We'll see about that!' Mrs Williams declared.

The next morning the three bullies were in the Headteacher's office.

'What have you got to say for yourselves?' Mr Beasely, the Headteacher, asked Richard, Mark and Simon.

'We were only playing… It was a bit of fun,' Simon told him.

'It is not fun if one of you doesn't enjoy the game or doesn't want to play, as with David,' Mr Beasely stated.

'We didn't know he wasn't having as much fun as we were,' protested Mark. 'He never said.'

'How do you account for his missing things? Where are they?'

'We can't help it if he loses things and forgets where he puts them,' piped Richard.

'Perhaps you'll be more co-operative when your parents arrive. I take a very dim view of bullying in any form and the thing about bullies is that they bully again and again throughout their lives unless someone puts a stop to it. Even wives and children. And they are so low they always pick on people weaker than themselves. Hardly fair, was it? Three to one? Weren't brave enough for one-to-one encounters?

'Not for one moment do I doubt David's word. You are going to have to earn the money to buy replacement clothes, bag and calculator for David unless they turn up tomorrow morning in pristine condition. I will discuss with your parents the length of your suspensions and what they intend to do about your behaviour. And even when it is all sorted out I shall have my eye on you all for any future trouble. If you're expecting references when you leave, you need to change your behaviour. Fast. Do I make myself clear?'

Discussion Sheet 13: We Were Only Playing

1. What would you have done in David's place when his bag was snatched from him?

2. (a) How would you react to being bullied in the long term?

   (b) What can you do to protect yourself from bullies?

3. Do you believe David's situation would have improved had he managed to hide his problem from his parents?

4. Do you think you should fight bullies yourself, get an older brother or sister to sort them out or go through official school channels?

5. Have you ever been a bully (including to a younger brother or sister) or been bullied? If so, why?

6. (a) How many emotions can you think of to describe how David might have felt?

   (b) How easy would it be for him to recover from the experience?

7. (a) Try and describe the sort of person you think a bully is.

   (b) Do female bullies bully differently to male bullies?

8. Why do children become bullies?

9. (a) Why do you think people become victims of bullying?

   (b) What effect does bullying have on them?

   (c) Are they programmed for life to be bullied, is it just chance, or does one experience shatter their confidence with people in the future, leaving them vulnerable to victimisation?

10. (a) Was the Headteacher of the school right? Do bullies never grow out of bullying?

    (b) Are their future families at risk?

    (c) Should they seek help themselves?

Leader Sheet 13: We Were Only Playing

1. **What would you have done in David's place when his bag was snatched from him?**

   (Personal response required.)

2. **(a) How would you react to being bullied in the longterm?**

   (Personal response required.)

   (b) What can you do to protect yourself from bullies?
   - You could try to avoid the bully whenever possible.
   - When confronted and threatened, inform the bully that you will tell on him or her if you are not left alone. Mean it and carry it through if necessary. (You could tell your teacher, your parents or guardians or the police.)
   - Try to avoid lonely places. For example, don't go to the toilets on your own if you feel unsafe or suspect the bully might be waiting for you there.
   - Try to get witnesses to anything that has happened to you at the bully's hands that will strengthen your case. Make people take you seriously.
   - Try to increase your confidence by becoming physically fit, learning to be assertive and learning confident body language. Practise behaving in a confident way.

3. **Do you believe David's situation would have improved had he managed to hide his problem from his parents?**

   No – it would have got worse because the boys would feel even more confident and powerful, knowing that David was too weak to tell on them. They would get more 'cocky' and do worse things.

4. **Do you think you should fight bullies yourself, get an older brother or sister to sort them out or go through official school channels?**
   - You might get hurt if you try to fight back yourself – unless you have a good chance of beating them. But when it's not one-to-one, there probably isn't much hope and it would give the

bullies a good excuse to hurt you even more. Also, fighting bullies does not stop them from bullying others. You really should talk to an adult about bullying behaviour.

- Getting an older brother or sister might help if they have the stature and the strength to overcome them – but it could go badly wrong if they couldn't and in such fights, people can get badly hurt, even killed. (What if one of the bullies had a knife, that he or she unexpectedly used on your brother or sister?)

- Going through official school channels would be best – but does the school have a strong anti-bullying policy? (If the bullying is racially linked, does the school have an anti-racist policy?) Some schools are better at dealing with bullies than others. They should get all parents involved and take a strong line of action with the bullies.

- If you were physically attacked, or threatened, as part of the bullying, you could go straight to the police.

5. **Have you ever been a bully (including to a younger brother or sister) or been bullied? If so, why?**

(Personal responses required.)

6. (a) **How many emotions can you think of to describe how David might have felt?**

David might have felt:

- alone
- angry
- ashamed
- bitter
- cowardly
- embarrassed
- friendless
- frustrated
- humiliated
- isolated
- powerless

- unwanted
- weak.

(b) How easy would it be for him to recover from the experience?

It might be difficult for him to recover from the experience. The longer the bullying has gone on, the greater the effects on the victim's self-esteem and self-confidence. He could become very shy and passive, feeling isolated and depressed. His schoolwork might suffer as he might develop problems in concentrating through stress. He might feel suicidal.

7. **(a) Try and describe the sort of person you think a bully is.**

A bully is someone who:

- likes to have power over others
- likes to make others do things he or she asks
- likes to frighten people
- likes to humiliate people
- likes to get his or her own way
- is probably bullied at home or lives with an aggressive parent
- needs help.

(b) Do female bullies bully differently to male bullies?

- Boy bullies are more likely to use physical threats with other boys – threatening to harm them if they don't do what they're told or give what the bully wants.
- Girl bullies are more likely to use social threats with other girls – that is, threatening not to be the person's friend any more or to start rumours about the person if he or she doesn't comply with their demands. They are more likely to make hurtful jokes and call people hurtful names. They can also get others to ignore the victim so that he or she she is effectively isolated from social support.

8. **Why do children become bullies?**

- Because they have a problem with their home life or upbringing that they cannot cope with. (Home stresses that children suffer personally, or see happen to another family member, include unemployment, divorce, alcoholism, bereavement, imprisonment and violence.)

- Because they have experienced ineffectual parenting where threats of punishment are not carried through, effectively rewarding them for negative behaviour. (Only when their parents are sufficiently riled is action taken and then it may be violent and extreme.)

- Because they want to have their own way, at any cost, and do not care who this might hurt.

- Because they have feelings that are not understood and needs that are not addressed, making them feel bitter and angry, so they take out their frustration on someone they see as weaker than themselves. Or the children might be victims of abuse and take out their hurt on others.

- Because they have not had a positive role model to copy and so do not know how to handle feelings of anger and frustration without resorting to violence or manipulation (social threats).

- Because they do not have high self-esteem and so need to prove themselves stronger than others and need to feel in control, by getting others to do what they want.

- They act aggressively to attract attention, feeling that negative attention is better than none.

- Because they have become involved with others who behave in anti-social ways and do it to be in with the group – like with a gang.

- They may be jealous of others who are richer, have more friends or greater talent than themselves.

9. (a) Why do you think people become victims of bullying?

- They are just unlucky to be in the wrong place at the wrong time.

- They display passive or timid body language so bullies see them as an easy target.

- They have little confidence so are not good at standing up for themselves.

- They are bullied at home and so accept their role as the down-trodden.

- They are perceived as being 'weak' in some way, such as not being good at sports.
- They do not wear the right clothes (unfashionable clothes or non-designer trainers).
- They are different to the majority in some way. This can be in the way they look (freckles, very thin, very fat, unfashionable hairstyle) or their ethnic origin, the way they speak or because they have some disability (wear glasses or a hearing aid, limp, have a speech impediment, use a wheelchair).
- Their parents or guardians are different in some way to the majority (over-protective, dress unusually, have a different accent, eccentric in some way).
- Their parents, guardians or other family members have particular problems that others have got to know about, such as alcoholism, drug addiction, imprisonment or multiple partners.
- They like attention so create a big fuss about small things and get noticed by people who are eager to take advantage of them.
- They are seen as 'swots' or have a special talent that is not accepted by the majority (for example, a boy being good at dancing instead of the stereotypically acceptable football or rugby).

(b) What effect does bullying have on them?

- They may remain socially passive, only speaking to those who speak to them first, never taking the initiative and not being the first to try to make a new friend.
- They may be easily intimidated.
- They may feel unable to cope.
- They may be very lonely, being rejected by their peers.
- They may become self-critical and self-hating, having very low self-esteem.
- They may become depressed and try to harm themselves.

(c) Are they programmed for life to be bullied, is it just chance, or does one experience shatter their confidence with people in the future, leaving them vulnerable to victimisation?

- Some people seem to be programmed for life – they are abused at home which lowers their self-esteem, they are bullied at school and may end up in an abusing relationship. It is as though they have accepted this as their lot. (For some people it can take years of violence and abuse within a partnership before they leave for good – if they ever do.)

- Some people are bullied by chance – they are not abused at home, are confident and display confident body language. Something about them catches the fancy of the bully – it may be a passing whim.

- One bad experience of being bullied can change a person, making him or her vulnerable to bullying in the future. Being bullied dents their confidence to the extent that their body language shows them to be timid people who can be taken advantage of – and bosses in the workplace often do bully or harass employees under their supervision.

10. (a) Was the Headteacher of the school right? Do bullies never grow out of bullying?

Yes, the Headteacher probably was right – unless bullies seek help. Without help, they may see no reason to change their behaviour, particularly if they find it gets them what they want. Small bullies can then grow into big bullies and become much harder to deal with (and much more dangerous).

(b) Are their future families at risk?

If bullying is a part of someone's nature, because he or she has been brought up in an abusive household, the bully has only had his or her parents or guardians as role models – and they are negative ones. The child may behave abusively towards his or her partner and children.

(c) Should they seek help themselves?

Yes, bullies should seek help – they can have happier and more fulfilling lives without the aggression and hate that builds up inside them. It might also stop them from going one step too far with the aggression and badly hurting someone or killing them. If bullying behaviour is allowed to continue, bullies' anti-social behaviour may lead to crime, spouse and child abuse, substance abuse and being able to socialise only with others who have similar behaviour, having alienated themselves from people who do not behave this way.

STORY 14: *Chicken!*

Richard and Simon saw the new boy at the newsagent's when they went to buy some drink and sweets. They nudged each other and decided to have some fun.

'Hi, Kenneth. Want to come for a walk with us? Get to know the area a bit better?'

Kenneth wanted to go straight home but knew he wasn't expected immediately. It would look as though he were afraid of them if he refused. They'd think him chicken.

'OK. But I can't be out long.' Kenneth thought that would give him the excuse to leave if he didn't like being with them. He wanted to make friends but there was something about these two he wasn't sure about. Maybe because they kept sniggering to each other as though they always had a private joke.

Richard and Simon took Kenneth through the local park and down an alley on to some wasteland. To one side of this there were bushes hiding the wire fencing that surrounded the railway track. Kenneth felt nervous.

Richard led the way and showed Kenneth where the fence had been cut, lifting up the free edge so that he could crawl through. 'Come on,' Richard said to Kenneth, motioning him to follow. Simon stood right behind him so Kenneth didn't have much choice.

'This is what we do,' explained Simon. 'We put coins on the track so that they get squashed when the train comes. Everyone in our gang has squashed coins. If you want to be with us, you must too.'

Kenneth felt sick. 'I think that's a stupid idea. I'm not going to risk...'

Richard and Simon began to make clucking noises. They were having great fun.

'I'll do it,' said Kenneth, 'but I still think it's a stupid idea.'

He walked toward the first track and laid down two coins.

'The next train comes from the other way – you need to put them on the second lot of tracks,' Simon shouted.

Kenneth sighed, picked up his coins, looked both ways and carefully stepped over the tracks. He put the coins down and stood well away from the track in the valley that side, listening to the hiss of the approaching train.

The train came and squashed the coins. Kenneth picked them up and took them back to show Richard and Simon.

'Great.' They laughed. 'Now,' said Richard, 'it's time for the next test. When the train this side comes round that bend, you start to run – across the tracks. If you're not quick enough...'

'I'm going. You're mad.'

'You're not going anywhere. All the new boys do this. It initiates them into the school. Everyone does it,' Simon lied. 'You can go when you've done it. Chicken.'

The train was coming and Kenneth started to run.

'Not yet!' Richard shouted, holding on to Kenneth's jumper. Only until after the train passed the bend did Richard let go. Kenneth ran, thinking he'd be pushed under if he didn't get away. But he was short of time.

'Look out!' Simon cried. Richard's hands covered his eyes.

The train passed and there was no sign of Kenneth. Nothing. The train must have taken him away. They ran.

Kenneth lay in fright for half an hour before he dared move. The dip in the valley had hidden his body and Richard and Simon had been too chicken to come and look. He swore. Never, ever would they do that to someone else and never, ever to him again. He knew the only way to stop them was to tell his parents and involve the police. He bet they'd be expelled too.

Discussion Sheet 14: Chicken!

1. Have you ever been called chicken? If so, why, and how did you feel about it?

2. Have you ever forced someone to do something he or she didn't want to? If so, why, and how did you do it?

3. What other games of 'Chicken' can you think of?

4. (a) Have you ever trespassed on railway property or areas fenced in for electricity substations?

(b) What are the dangers of these places?

5. Should Kenneth have gone with Richard and Simon, as he didn't really know them? Why?

6. What would you have done if you were Kenneth once he'd found out what the boys expected of him?

7. Do you think this story showed a form of bullying? Give reasons for your answer.

8. Why do you think Richard and Simon forced Kenneth to play 'Chicken'? Think of as many reasons as you can.

9. Should Kenneth have reported Richard and Simon to the police? Why?

10. What happens if actions like those of Richard and Simon go unreported?

Leader Sheet 14: Chicken!

1. *Have you ever been called chicken? If so, why, and how did you feel about it?*

   (Personal responses required.)

2. *Have you ever forced someone to do something he or she didn't want to? If so, why, and how did you do it?*

   (Personal responses required.)

3. *What other games of 'Chicken' can you think of?*

   - Running across a busy road or crossing directly in front of an oncoming car or lorry.
   - Being dared to do dangerous things such as climb onto a roof or cross a fast-flowing river when you can't swim.

4. *(a) Have you ever trespassed on railway property or areas fenced in for electricity substations?*

   (Personal response required.)

   (b) What are the dangers of these places?

   Railways:

   - You can get electrocuted.
   - You can be run over by a train.
   - You can trip up and be injured so that you lie across the path of an oncoming train.

   Electricity substations:

   - You don't have to touch the equipment to get electrocuted. The voltage is so high that electricity can easily jump across a gap and go through you, killing you.

5. *Should Kenneth have gone with Richard and Simon as he didn't really know them? Why?*

   No, as there was something about them he didn't trust. He should have listened to his gut instincts. The fact that they kept giggling should have warned him more strongly. He could have refused to go with them from the start without much loss of face. And pride loses its importance when it's measured against personal safety. Children might think that other children are safe, as parents and guardians warn their children about wicked adults, not children. However, this is not always the case. (The toddler, James Bulger, was abducted and killed by two boys.)

6. What would you have done if you were Kenneth once he'd found out what the boys expected of him?

(Personal response required.)

7. Do you think this story showed a form of bullying? Give reasons for your answer.

Yes. Richard and Simon had intimidated Kenneth and had forced him to do something against his will. They had also forced him to do something that could have cost him his life. They were the cowards, two close friends against one newcomer.

8. Why do you think Richard and Simon forced Kenneth to play 'Chicken'? Think of as many reasons as you can.

- It made them feel powerful.
- They had someone who would do whatever they asked.
- They knew Kenneth was vulnerable because he was new and wouldn't know if they were lying.
- They liked to see Kenneth squirm.
- They were bored and used Kenneth for their entertainment.
- They thought of the fun they would have at school telling other friends about it.
- They liked playing dangerous games.
- They were bullies and enjoyed bullying others.

9. Should Kenneth have reported Richard and Simon to the police? Why?

Yes. If the police weren't told, Richard and Simon might force someone else to run across the tracks and this next time, the person might die. Only the police could stop it from happening again, by showing them, their parents or guardians and their teachers how foolhardy the boys had been. Bullies do not tend to stop themselves, they keep on terrorising people. Also, they'd had a warning in the last story, yet still chose to carry on. It's time they took responsibility for their actions.

10. What happens if actions like those of Richard and Simon go unreported?

- The bullies might go on to do worse things because they know they can get away with it.
- They can become more dangerous and can ruin their victims' lives.
- Other people might be encouraged to become bullies if they see others get away with it.
- Some fully-grown adults have needed counselling because of the effects bullying has had on them – it is not something the victim easily gets over, the memory and the feelings can remain with the person.

No one has a right to affect someone else's life in a negative way for his or her own amusement.

STORY 15: *Honesty Policy*

Vicky ran to answer the phone. 'If it's Nigel, I'm not in,' her brother, Sean, called. 'I arranged to go to Paul's today and he wasn't asked.'

'Hello?'

'Is Sean there please?'

'Who is it?'

'Nigel.'

'He says he's not in,' Vicky told him and hung up.

Sean was listening on the stairs. 'You were supposed to say I wasn't in, not that I *said* I wasn't!'

'But that would have been a lie!' Vicky sanctimoniously told him.

Cassie came home with some shortbread she made at school. 'It's for you, Mum,' she said proudly.

'But Mum hates shortbread,' Vicky told her. Cassie's face fell.

'Thank you, Cassie. That was very kind of you,' their Mum said.

'But you don't like it,' Cassie burst out as she ran upstairs crying.

'Honestly, Vicky, I don't know what to do with you sometimes. That was very unkind.'

Sean was looking after Vicky while their Mum was out with Cassie and took her to Nigel's house with him. Vicky saw a photograph of Nigel on the mantelpiece and picked it up. 'You've got more spots now than you have here,' she commented. Nigel blushed. Sean raised his eyes to the ceiling. He hated taking his little sister anywhere – she was always putting her foot in it. Anyone would think she did it on purpose.

Vicky and her mum went to visit Miranda's family as her uncle had just died. 'I bet you're glad now,' Vicky told Miranda in front of everyone. 'You never did like him did you?'

Miranda was stunned and her mother looked at Vicky tearfully. Vicky's mum wanted to run out and pretend what her daughter had said had never happened.

'What do you think?' Vicky's mum asked, twirling in front of the mirror, showing her new dress off.

'The colour's revolting and it's too short on you. But I like the neckline.'

'Thanks. I might have known I shouldn't ask you.' Vicky's mum quickly changed back into her ordinary clothes. She returned the dress the following day.

'Vicky, will you stop talking while I'm trying to explain what you're all to do.'

'It wasn't me Miss, it was Miranda.' The rest of the pupils turned and hissed at her.

'That's enough, class,' the teacher told them. Vicky really exasperated her. She'd never known a child so unlikeable.

One lunchtime, Vicky and Miranda were messing about in the corridor, throwing each other's books around. Miranda picked up Vicky's library book and flung it across the corridor in retaliation for her books being strewn everywhere. They were having great fun until Miranda's throw sent the book smashing into the fire alarm and set it going. The bell shrilled loudly as they gathered up their things and rushed out with everyone else.

Mr Beasley, the Headteacher, threatened a whole school detention if the culprit didn't own up by the morning. But Vicky didn't wait that long.

'Yes, Victoria, what can I do for you?' Mr Beasley asked as his secretary showed her in.

'It's about the fire alarm, sir.'

'Yes?'

'I started it off. I was angry and threw a book and it hit the alarm accidentally.'

Mr Beasley looked at her file and believed her. He was pleased that he didn't have to go to any great lengths to get someone to own up. It made his life easier. 'I'm afraid I shall have to make an example of you so that the rest of the school doesn't think they can get away with "accidentally" setting off the fire alarm. You're suspended for two days.'

Telling the truth hadn't worked out for Vicky. Everyone said, 'Honesty is the Best Policy' – but who actually believed it? By owning up to Miranda's mistake, Vicky had repaid the pain she'd caused her friend. She was done with telling the truth. It wasn't what people wanted to hear.

Discussion Sheet 15: Honesty Policy

1. (a) What is tact?

    (b) Is it dishonest?

2. Give alternative acceptable comments Vicky could have made in each circumstance except the last.

3. Did any of Vicky's comments need to be honest? Why?

4. How would you react to someone asking your advice about clothes? Would you tell them they looked great and let them look a fool if they didn't, or would you be totally honest or try to 'sweeten the pill'?

5. Have you been asked by a family member to lie for them? Did your parents or guardians approve of this? Is this contrary to how they brought you up? Does it confuse you?

6. (a) As Vicky had never been known to tell a lie, the Headteacher immediately believed her. Was it stupid of her to take the blame in this instance?

    (b) What future consequences may make her regret this act?

7. In Aesop's fables, the boy who 'cried wolf' was so used to lying that in the end no one believed a word he said. How do you want yourself to be perceived? Why?

8. (a) Under what circumstances would you, or do you, lie? Why?

    (b) What are the dangers if you habitually lie?

9. (a) What is a 'white lie'?

    (b) Why is the colour white used in this context?

    (c) Do you find it easy to distinguish between lies that matter and lies that don't?

    (d) Give examples of each.

10. (a) When someone asks you to be totally honest, does he or she always mean it?

    (b) Can your self-esteem take undiluted criticism?

    (c) How can you strike a good balance so that your judgements are valued but you do not crush a person's feelings?

Leader Sheet 15: Honesty Policy

---

1. (a) What is tact?

Tact is about saying the right things and not giving offence to people.

(b) Is it dishonest?

It is dishonest if it is taken to extremes, such as saying you love something when you don't. It would be better to say 'I preferred the other one' or 'I'm not sure about the colour' – concentrating on one part rather than the whole thing.

2. Give alternative acceptable comments Vicky could have made in each circumstance except the last.

Phone call: 'I'm not sure where he is. Can I ask my Mum?' – or just lie as you were asked. More damage was done on both sides by not lying. Her brother wouldn't feel so embarrassed and his friend wouldn't feel so hurt.

Shortbread: 'What a lovely surprise for Mum.' Vicky could leave the responsibility of the shortbread to her mum. If her mum really couldn't stand shortbread, she could tell Cassie she'd save it for later, when she relaxes in front of the television after her children are in bed.

Photograph: No comment was needed. Vicky should have kept the thought to herself. If she wanted to ask a question, she could have asked something neutral such as 'How old were you when this was taken?'

Funeral: Again, Vicky should have kept quiet. If she wanted to say something to her friend, she could have said, 'Are you OK?'

Mum's dress: 'I'm not sure that the colour does anything for you, but it's a pretty neckline.' Her mum may have thought over what Vicky had said about the colour later, and decided not to keep the dress, without being told outright she had bad taste.

In class: Vicky wasn't in huge trouble about the talking. She could have let that one go and say, 'Sorry Miss', or she could have given a body language gesture of surprise – that of opening her mouth as though about to protest her innocence. The teacher may have got the message without it being obvious to everyone.

3. *Did any of Vicky's comments need to be honest? Why?*

The comment about her mum's dress had to be honest. If she'd lied about that, her mum might look stupid in public, thinking it really did suit her. Plus her mum would have wasted her money. It isn't kind to let people make fools of themselves.

4. *How would you react to someone asking your advice about clothes? Would you tell them they looked great and let them look a fool if they didn't, or would you be totally honest or try to 'sweeten the pill'?*

(Personal response required.)

5. *Have you been asked by a family member to lie for them? Did your parents or guardians approve of this? Is this contrary to how they brought you up? Does it confuse you?*

(Personal responses required.)

6. (a) *As Vicky had never been known to tell a lie, the Headteacher immediately believed her. Was it stupid of her to take the blame in this instance?*

- There was no need for her to take the blame. It had been an accident and her friend Miranda might not have got into too much trouble. However, owning up to it did make amends with Miranda. (However, Miranda may have preferred to take responsibility rather than face feeling guilty that Vicky took the blame.)

(b) *What future consequences may make her regret this act?*

- She may regret it once her parents know she'd been suspended. Suspension is a rather harsh disciplinary measure for an accident but the Headteacher obviously didn't want it to catch on as a fun thing to do so chose to make an example of her.

- She may also regret it when she comes to needing a reference – it would go down on her school records that she'd been suspended, and the referee may not be so gushing about her positive attributes.

7. *In Aesop's fables, the boy who 'cried wolf' was so used to lying that in the end no one believed a word he said. How do you want yourself to be perceived? Why?*

(Personal response required.)

8. *(a) Under what circumstances would you, or do you, lie? Why?*

- To protect yourself – you can go to any lengths to keep yourself safe from harm.

- To protect a friend – you might do this for minor things and it is natural that you should want to. However, if someone has committed a bad crime he or she should take responsibility for it. If not, the person may repeat it and then you would have to take some of the blame because you allowed it to continue.

- If the issue is of no importance to anyone. For example, if you are asked how you are and you feel upset because you have had a bad day, you still might say 'Fine', because you don't want to have to explain to someone you're not close to.

- To give someone some space. For example, if you knew that your friend was upset and needed some time alone, and you were asked by another where he or she was – you might say you didn't know so that your friend could have more undisturbed time.

- To get out of trouble – denying something when you have done it.

(b) What are the dangers if you habitually lie?

- No one believes you when you are telling the truth.
- People might think that, because you lie, you also do other negative things such as steal or break rules.

9. *(a) What is a 'white lie'?*

A white lie is a small, harmless lie that doesn't hurt anyone.

(b) Why is the colour white used in this context?

Probably because it is the opposite of black and the colour black has been given negative connotations. (For example: blackleg – one who refuses to join a trade union or breaks other's strikes by working for that employer; blacklist – a list of people who have done wrong or who will be treated in a negative way; blackmail – extorting money using threats; Black Monday – the description given to the day in 1987 when the world stock market crash began; Black Thursday when, in 1929, the US Wall Street stock market crashed.)

(c) Do you find it easy to distinguish between lies that matter and lies that don't?

(Personal response required.)

(d) Give examples of each.

Examples of white lies:

- If you've been taken out for the day and you're asked if you enjoyed it. It would be rude to say, 'no', so you'd say 'yes', even if you hadn't.

- You don't feel well when you're out with a friend. You don't want to spoil her fun so when she asks if you are OK, you say 'yes'.

- A neighbour has an urgent problem and has to pop out. She asks if you wouldn't mind going round to look after her toddler for half and hour and says, 'You're not busy are you? Is it OK?' You answer, 'Fine, no problem' because it would be unkind to refuse someone in need even if you do have a stack of homework to do.

Examples of lies that matter:

- If you were a witness to an incident where someone got hurt but you say you saw nothing, the victim is then victim twice over. The victim deserves to have the culprit brought to justice if it is within someone's power to make it happen.

- If you did something that was wrong and you lie when asked about it, you are not accepting responsibility for your actions. The person may still suspect it was you and would not respect you for lying.

- Lying to protect someone else by supplying an alibi.
- Lying to your partner saying you love him or her when you don't. He or she has a right to know before, for example, a commitment of marriage is made.

10. (a) When someone asks you to be totally honest, does he or she always mean it?

No, often they don't. They mean will you say it in a tactful, watered down way that won't hurt their feelings too much and will you also tell them what they could do to put it right. (Positive criticism.)

(b) Can your self-esteem take undiluted criticism?

(Personal response required.)

(c) How can you strike a good balance so that your judgements are valued but you do not crush a person's feelings?

Pick on a couple of things that stand out as being needed to be spoken about, and brush over the rest or ignore it. Being totally blunt can crush a person's confidence. You could also tentatively suggest he or she seeks a second opinion – say that you don't know much about whatever they have asked you about.

STORY 16: *Painful Puberty*

My name's Paul and I'm not too happy. I'm spotty and have started to grow silly thin hairs on my face – not enough to start shaving because there aren't enough of them, but enough to look stupid.

My penis and testes have got much bigger and I like to keep looking at them to check they're just as big as everyone else's. I also get turned on all the time – at the slightest thing. I get worried that people will notice and tease me about it. A girl only has to brush against me and it's standing up hard.

As for my sheets, I wish Mum would let me do my own washing now. I have wet dreams and often wake up in a sticky mess from ejaculating in bed. I feel like a child that can't control himself.

I enjoy playing with myself too – but feel guilty. I often wonder if any of my friends masturbate but if one of them asked me, I'd deny it. I think of sex and girls all the time – I can't help it. We talk about sex at school but only among the boys – girls seem interested in romance more than sex and anyway, it's man talk.

My breasts look bigger too. Mum says it's all right, it's just temporary because of my hormone changes.

The worst thing of all is my voice. It's gone deep which I like. It makes me feel like a real man. But every so often it squeaks back to what it was and everyone laughs at me. Then I blush.

My name's Mary and I'm not very happy. I keep crying. At the slightest thing. My older brother and my parents often tease me and I get very upset about it. I spend much of my time alone in my room. I don't know how to deal with my feelings. They overwhelm me and I don't know what's wrong with me. I'm so irritable with everyone including myself.

I look in the mirror and hate what I see – a spotty girl with a podgy tummy and almost flat chest. My breasts have been desperately sore for a long while now and I'm scared that someone will run into me when I'm in the schoolyard or in crowds, they hurt so much. My knickers are often stained with this sticky clear stuff that keeps coming out. And my first period started yesterday.

It doesn't hurt at all but I'm worried that I'll leak. Mum gave me these thick pads to wear but they move when I walk and when I feel a load of blood come out I think it'll overflow down my legs. And it's hard to stay clean – I'm worried people might smell me when I've been to the toilet.

I'm quite pleased that I've got my period at last – most of my friends already have theirs and I felt as though I was still very much a child not having them too.

I'd like to have my first bra too but Mum says I don't need one yet as there's not much there.

I get teased at school. There's this teacher I really like – Miss Atkinson – and every time I talk to her or have to answer a question I go bright red. I blush at anything. Well, my friends have noticed that it always happens with her – even if she just passes me in the corridor and they say I fancy her but I don't. They think I'm a lesbian but I'm not. Am I?

Discussion Sheet 16: Painful Puberty

1. What changes do you like about puberty. Why?

2. What changes do you dislike about puberty. Why?

3. What things (if any) have worried you?

4. Can you talk about puberty or sex with an adult or older brother or sister? If not, why not?

5. (a) Can you think of reasons why people masturbate and reasons why they don't?

   (b) Have any adults or other people made their view on masturbation known to you?

   (c) Has it affected how you view it? (This question is *not* asking you if you do masturbate.)

6. Do you feel you own your own body and have a right to touch and look at any part or do you feel this is not allowed? If so, what or who gave you this no touch, no look feeling and how? (To get to know your body it is a

good idea to hold a mirror between your legs so that you can see what is part of you.)

7. (a) Are you unsure of your sexuality? (Be honest with yourself, even if you do not wish to talk about it with others.)

    (b) Mary worries she may be a lesbian. What do you think?

    (c) If you were friends with Mary, would it make any difference if Mary were a lesbian? Why?

    (d) Who gave you this viewpoint or is it purely your own?

8. Do your parents or guardians make allowances for your mood swings in puberty? If not, can you explain your feelings to them?

9. What do you feel about the opposite sex? How do you think they feel about your sex?

10. (a) As a culture, the British often seem obsessed with hygiene and smell. What is a good cleansing programme?

    (b) Why is it not good to go over the top about body cleanliness?

Leader Sheet 16: Painful Puberty

1. **What changes do you like about puberty. Why?**

   Girls: Developing breasts and hips. They make you feel feminine and like a woman.

   Boys: Having a larger penis, having a deep voice, having hairs on your face. They make you feel like a man. Erections are nice too, but can be very embarrassing.

2. **What changes do you dislike about puberty. Why?**

   Both: Sweating more. Having spots, greasy hair and skin.

   Girls: Having periods because they are messy and a nuisance.
   The mood swings get you down – being so tearful and grumpy makes you feel miserable.
   Having damp knickers from discharge.

   Boys: Having wet dreams – although they're nice, they're very embarrassing and you don't want your mum to see your sheets.
   The squeaks your voice makes when it switches pitch makes you feel silly.

3. **What things (if any) have worried you?**

   Many girls worry about childbirth and labour pains. Many other worries are due to embarrassment – girls might fear their genitals aren't normal, yet are too shy to ask a doctor to check for them. Boys might worry that their penises are small.
   A worry for girls using tampons is the rare possibility of Toxic Shock Syndrome (TSS). This is a type of blood poisoning that can make you very ill very quickly, half of the cases being tampon-related. The risk can be reduced by using the lowest suitable absorbency tampon for your period flow, changing it regularly, and having stretches where it is not used at all (such as overnight).

4. **Can you talk about puberty or sex with an adult or older brother or sister? If not, why not?**

   (Personal responses required.)

5. **(a)** *Can you think of reasons why people masturbate and reasons why they don't?*

Reasons for masturbating:

- It can be very pleasurable.
- You learn about your own body.
- It can release tension.
- There's no chance of you getting pregnant or developing a sexually transmitted disease.
- For some people, it is the only way they can achieve orgasm.
- Some people do not have a partner, so would have unfulfilled sex lives if they did not masturbate at all.
- Mutual masturbation is a safe way of having sex with a partner. (There is no risk of pregnancy or of developing a sexually transmitted disease.)

Reasons against masturbating:

- For very religious people, the guilt they feel afterwards is not worth the experience. (Catholic priests have to confess to their priest on every occasion they succumb to masturbation. They also preach that their congregation should do the same.)
- Some people feel bad about themselves, believing it is not right to 'have sex with oneself'.

(b) *Have any adults or other people made their view on masturbation known to you?*

Some religions teach that masturbation is wrong. There are some old wives' tales about turning blind if the person masturbates which is obviously untrue. Parents and guardians don't tend to talk about masturbation to their children, it's a 'taboo' subject. They probably hope their child doesn't know about it. There are plenty of jokes about masturbation but it's a little discussed subject, even among friends.

(c) *Has it affected how you view it? (This question is __not__ asking you if you do masturbate.)*

(Personal response required.)

6. *Do you feel you own your own body and have a right to touch and look at any part or do you feel this is not allowed? If so, what or who gave you this no touch, no look feeling and how? (To get to know your body it is a good idea to hold a mirror between your legs so that you can see what is part of you.)*

Many parents and guardians bring up their children to think that their body (or genital area) is dirty and that they should not look at it. Years ago, modest women would not see their own bodies, getting undressed underneath a long night-gown. Some men would not see their wives naked.

Parents and guardians are often too embarrassed to discuss bodies with their children and consider sex 'dirty' or unmentionable. This can give their children bad feelings about themselves and their bodies. It may also make it harder for these people to 'let go' when they are having sex and so they get little pleasure from the act, instead of it being a loving and intimate experience.

7. *(a) Are you unsure of your sexuality? (Be honest with yourself, even if you do not wish to talk about it with others.)*

(Personal response required.)

(b) Mary worries she may be a lesbian. What do you think?

Many girls admire female teachers to the extent of blushing about it – having strong role models is a natural part of growing up. This does not necessarily make her a lesbian.

(c) If you were friends with Mary, would it make any difference if Mary were a lesbian? Why?

Yes: You'd be worried that she might fancy you. (However, homosexuals don't fancy everyone of the same sex just as heterosexuals don't fancy everyone of the opposite sex.)

No: You'd be curious to find out how she feels and how she sees the world but it would make no difference to your friendship with her. It could deepen the relationship, reaching a new understanding of each other instead of hiding what's going on.

(d) Who gave you this viewpoint or is it purely your own?

(Personal response required.)

8. *Do your parents or guardians make allowances for your mood swings in puberty? If not, can you explain your feelings to them?*

(Personal responses required.)

9. *What do you feel about the opposite sex? How do you think they feel about your sex?*

(Personal responses required.)

10. *(a) As a culture, the British often seem obsessed with hygiene and smell. What is a good cleansing programme?*

- Bath or shower either every other day or once a day.

- Once you hit puberty you sweat more, so use an anti-perspirant after your shower and before you get dressed for the day.

- Hair gets greasier and needs to be washed more often. However, if it is washed every day, it can become greasier still. Try every other day, or less if your hair is dry.

- Have clean underwear and socks every day.

- Check shirt/top armpits for stains and smell. If they look and smell clean, you can get away with wearing them for a second day. If in doubt, have fresh clothes. Smell jeans and trousers too. Wash them when you can detect body smell on them.

(b) Why is it not good to go over the top about body cleanliness?

Over the top washing can destroy the healthy bugs on your body and make you susceptible to thrush. Also, if you wash your hair too often it can make it oilier still.

STORY 17: Nightmare

'Come in, Peter. Steven's in the lounge. We're on our way out so we'll see you later.'

'OK, Mrs Roberts. Have a nice time.'

Steve's parents left to go to the cinema. He and Pete were babysitting Steve's sister. It was a regular event.

'Hi,' Pete said.

'Hi. Have you got it?' Steve asked.

'Yo!' Pete brandished the video after fishing it out of his bag. 'No probs.' He sank on to the settee, put his feet on the coffee table and passed the video to his friend.

Steve put it on and they began to watch the trailers, bags of crisps in hand. The volume was on quite high and Steve switched off the main light leaving only a table lamp to give the room a glow. The scene was set...

Eight-year-old Vanessa tiptoed halfway down the stairs. She couldn't resist the noise any longer and wanted to see what they were watching. The sitting-room door was open and she could see the television screen while sitting on the stairs.

An hour later Vanessa was riveted. She couldn't have moved even if she'd wanted to, as she was so scared. Scared of the unimaginable... All she could do was watch with eyes open wide, fingers in her mouth.

The following week Mrs Roberts noticed that Vanessa had become very quiet and withdrawn. She kept waking at night, lashing her arms about and moaning. In the daytime, she followed her everywhere as if afraid to be alone. She jumped at the slightest noise, was reluctant to go to bed and had to have the landing light on all night.

'Vanessa, I know there's something wrong. Please tell me what's bothering you.'

They were in the kitchen and Mrs Roberts was preparing some chicken breasts, skinning them with a knife. Vanessa watched with fascinated horror.

Her mother noticed that she seemed rather preoccupied with the knife. She stopped what she was doing.

'I want you to tell me. Now. You're not leaving this room until you do.'

After Steve had gone to sleep that night, Mrs Roberts put on a woolly hat and scarf, crept into his room and picked up a toy knife. Leaning over Steve, she gently shook him.

'Aah!!' As soon as he'd opened his eyes he screamed and jumped out of bed, yelling incoherently. His mother switched on the light.

'What the hell did you do that for?' he demanded, heart pounding.

'What the hell have you done to my daughter?' she replied angrily. 'And, by the looks of things, to yourself? And don't swear at me!'

'I don't know what you mean,' Steve faltered.

'I know all about the video. Vanessa told me. After a week of nightmares!'

'I didn't know she saw it. I thought she was in bed.'

'But you didn't check! Now you listen to me...' she took a deep breath. 'In future when Peter comes here, he's to show me what he has in his bag. And his jacket pockets. You are not to go to his house at all until I feel sure I can trust you not to look at any more video-nasties. And I'm about to ring his mother to see if she knew about it. And I bet this wasn't the first time?'

Steve hung his head. It hadn't been. Damn Vanessa!

'I am very, very angry. Goodness knows how long it will take Vanessa to get over this – or you if you're honest about it. It is not natural to watch such utterly SICK films!'

Discussion Sheet 17: Nightmare

1. Do you watch films with a rating higher than your age? If so, how have you managed to see them? Have you ever been refused a film in a video shop because they suspect you are under age?

2. Why do films have ratings?

3. If you have watched horror, violent or sexually explicit films what effect, if any, have they had? (Be honest.) Did you enjoy them? Did you consider any of them 'sick'?

4. (a) Why is there a demand for shocking, high-impact films?

   (b) They are so much more vivid and gory than, say, 10 or 20 years ago – are we so desensitised to the horrors of things like murder and torture that we need worse things to thrill us?

5. Have you ever had dreams affected by what you have watched? Has your behaviour ever altered because of it?

6. Do your parents or guardians censor what you watch? How do you feel about this?

7. One form of child abuse is not protecting children from unnecessary suffering. Do you think that if you are allowed to watch 'nasty' films you are being abused?

8. At the age of 16 you can legally smoke, have sex (in mainland Britain), get married and work full-time. Do you object to the fact that you are expected to wait until you are 18 to watch some films?

9. (a) Do you think that filmmakers ought to cut down on the violent or disturbing films they make?

   (b) What is your view on violent computer games?

10. The toddler James Bulger was abducted, tortured and killed by two young boys. They had enacted some of the scenes they had seen in a film. Psychologists now agree that watching video-nasties affects people's behaviour, especially that of younger viewers. How could we improve our society and make it a more caring one, respecting life?

Leader Sheet 17: Nightmare

1. *Do you watch films with a rating higher than your age? If so, how have you managed to see them? Have you ever been refused a film in a video shop because they suspect you are under age?*

   (Personal responses required.)

2. *Why do films have ratings?*

   To protect the viewer, and to inform parents and guardians that the film may contain unsuitable footage for their particular child.

3. *If you have watched horror, violent or sexually explicit films what effect, if any, have they had? (Be honest.) Did you enjoy them? Did you consider any of them 'sick'?*

   (Personal responses required.)

4. *(a) Why is there a demand for shocking, high-impact films?*

   Special effects have become more sophisticated so the thrills and scares we get from films now have more impact. Some people like to be scared by a film and look for the scariest around.

   (b) They are so much more vivid and gory than, say, 10 or 20 years ago – are we so desensitised to the horrors of things like murder and torture that we need worse things to thrill us?

   People who have already seen many films do get bored and desensitised, and are on the lookout for newer and more involving films. Those who like horror films want the experience to get scarier. Film producers are in competition to show off their talents for special effects and high-impact films.

5. *Have you ever had dreams affected by what you have watched? Has your behaviour ever altered because of it?*

   (Personal responses required.)

6. *Do your parents or guardians censor what you watch? How do you feel about this?*

   (Personal responses required.)

7. *One form of child abuse is not protecting children from unnecessary suffering. Do you think that if you are allowed to watch 'nasty' films you are being abused?*

- Part of a parent's or guardian's duty to his or her children is to protect them and keep them safe. By introducing them to a world of terror, they fail to do this.

- Children should not be presented with emotional material inappropriate to their age group. It may involve them too deeply and they might find it harder to think of the film as fiction – they may get stuck in the feelings that the film provoked just as children in role-play can get carried away with their role.

- The ways video-nasties affect children are not yet fully understood. But it has been reported in the news that children have behaved brutally after having seen disturbing films.

8. *At the age of 16 you can legally smoke, have sex (in mainland Britain), get married and work full-time. Do you object to the fact that you are expected to wait until you are 18 to watch some films?*

Yes: When you're 16, you're basically an adult. If you're legally in a sexual relationship you should be able to watch sexy films as you're already 'in the know'.

Everyone's heard loads of swearing by the time they are 16 – so what does it matter if there's swearing on a film? You're old enough to decide your own behaviour and the way you talk. You won't be influenced by a film.

By the time you're 16, you know that the violence you see on screen is make-believe. Why wait another two years?

No: The film boards must have good reason to think that the material is unsuitable for you and may harm you psychologically.

You don't mind not watching 18 films as you hate seeing any violence. Even when you are 18, you won't watch films with an 18 certificate. They're too nasty.

9. **(a) Do you think that filmmakers ought to cut down on the violent or disturbing films they make?**

Yes: It's not necessary to portray such evil and wickedness. You feel your world is a less safe place now than it used to be and blame much on the media.

When children do copycat crimes of things they've seen at the cinema, it's really sick.

Filmmakers have a responsibility to the public. They are creating psychological disturbances in some people and encouraging others to commit crimes.

No: People don't have to watch it if they don't like it. It's wrong to take away the enjoyment of the majority just because of a few that can't stomach it.

(b) What is your view on violent computer games?

- These may be considered worse than watching films because, with the games, you are actually taking part in a struggle and are interacting with the game. You take on a role that might involve repeated killing. It possibly creates more violence.

- Unlike films, where you might see the film once or twice (unless you have become obsessed with it), you play computer games again and again and try to improve your score – and perhaps to do this you might have to become more and more ruthless.

10. The toddler James Bulger was abducted, tortured and killed by two young boys. They had enacted some of the scenes they had seen in a film. Psychologists now agree that watching video-nasties affects people's behaviour, especially that of younger viewers. How could we improve our society and make it a more caring one, respecting life?

- Watch more positive films, showing people caring about one another instead of killing.

- If a film has to be violent, the violence could be implied – that is, no special effects of seeing someone's head sliced off, or blood spurting from a fatal chest wound.

- Protect younger children from some of the nastier side of life – such as abductions and murders (although this does not mean keeping them ignorant of how to keep themselves safe).

- Ban all violent films and games. Is violence something to use as entertainment?

- Have some kind of threshold beyond which filmmakers cannot go, to keep more of the detail and horror out of films.

- Produce more family films, so that the whole family can sit down together to enjoy a film.

- Discuss violent events that have happened in real life, on a television soap or on film in schools, to re-sensitise children and get them to understand, for example, the devastation a parent feels when their child is murdered. How do those parents whose children have been gunned down en masse in school feel? How would they feel, confronted by a gunman or a boy with a gun? (So far, such incidents have only occurred with men.)

STORY 18: I Fell Down the Stairs

'Morning girls. All changed?' The games teacher, Miss Flaherty, breezed into the changing rooms.

'Please Miss, I don't feel well,' Polly told her.

'What's the matter this time?'

'My stomach hurts.'

'What's that from, do you think?' Miss Flaherty waited for an answer but Polly just looked down. 'The fresh air might do you good. Hurry up and get changed, please.'

'But I feel sick too. Dreadfully sick.'

'And when did this start?' Miss Flaherty asked with disbelief. 'This morning? Five minutes ago? Look, this happens too often, Polly. Get changed quickly and don't keep the rest of the girls waiting.'

Polly didn't move.

'NOW!'

Polly took her kit and headed towards the toilets.

'Polly, we're all female. Stay where I can see you so that I don't forget you're joining us for netball this week.' Miss Flaherty was sarcastic.

Slowly, Polly undressed and by now all the girls had finished changing and were watching her.

As Miss Flaherty began to collect the watches and other valuables, Polly's friend gasped. Miss Flaherty turned back and saw Polly's arms. They were covered in purple bruises.

'Right girls, into the schoolyard and run round three times to warm up. Quickly!'

Polly covered up her arms and sat down, not knowing whether to feel glad or scared.

Miss Flaherty sat down next to her. 'How did you get those bruises, Polly?' she asked gently.

Polly shrugged.

'Marks don't get there by themselves, Polly, and I doubt very much that they are self-inflicted. Has it been going on long?' Polly quietly started to cry, but when Miss Flaherty put her arm around her she flinched and moved away. She didn't like people to touch her. 'I can't leave the girls on their own for much longer. Come to my office and I'll ring for Miss O'Connor to come and fetch you. She'll take over. And don't worry. It's all for the best. You should have said something long ago, you poor thing.'

Miss O'Connor put down the phone and addressed Polly. 'I've just phoned Social Services and I've informed the Head. He's phoning your mother to ask her to come in. A police officer will be coming too.'

'What's going to happen?' Polly asked.

'I'm not sure. We'll have to see what your mother has to say – and what the lady from Social Services thinks. It's not up to me. However, if she thinks you might be at risk, she may find somewhere else for you to stay until things get cleared up.'

Polly began to cry again. All her pent-up emotion was being released and she was very frightened.

'Would you like to talk about it to me?'

'You've got it wrong,' Polly declared. 'I fell down the stairs. It's nothing to do with my mum.'

'Your mum?'

Polly bit her lip.

'Polly, if that's so, why are you crying and why did you try to hide your body by not doing games? Look, there's no point in shielding whoever is responsible because it won't stop unless you have help. And a doctor will probably examine you to see whether your injuries can be explained by anything else other than abuse. For your own safety, you must tell the truth, Polly. However much it hurts. Even when you love someone, there are times when you must stop protecting bad things that they do. Whoever did it needs help too.'

Discussion Sheet 18: I Fell Down the Stairs

1. Why had Polly missed so many games lessons?

2. (a) What do you think Polly's everyday life was like?

(b) How do you think she felt when she woke up in the mornings?

3. Who do you think is most likely to be responsible for Polly's injuries and why?

4. Is it possible or likely that anyone else in the family was at risk too?

5. Suggest reasons why Polly tried to hide the fact that she was being abused.

6. Give as many examples as you can about ways in which a child can be abused.

7. What would you do if you were being abused? (If you really have been abused you may not wish to talk about it in front of others.) Is that the best way of dealing with the problem?

8. How would you feel if you were abused? Would you feel, in any way, that you deserved it?

9. (a) People can suffer years of abuse from their partner without seeking help. Why do abusers get away with it so often?

   (b) Why do their partners protect them?

10. (a) What do you think will happen to Polly's family in the long term?

    (b) How might the intervention change their lives?

    (c) Would Polly feel guilty about the part she had played in this?

Leader Sheet 18: I Fell Down the Stairs

1. ***Why had Polly missed so many games lessons?***

   She hadn't wanted anyone to see her body when she got changed. She wanted to hide her bruises as she knew she wouldn't be able to explain them.

2. ***(a) What do you think Polly's everyday life was like?***

   Polly probably lived in fear, never knowing when the next blow would come or why. She probably tried to be desperately careful about everything she did or said so she wouldn't upset or annoy the person who was abusing her.

   (b) How do you think she felt when she woke up in the mornings?

   She probably dreaded the day ahead. She must have felt very lonely, having no one to confide in about her troubles and being isolated from the care of her parents, as one or both were hurting her. She may have also had one of her parents abused by the other and had to cope with witnessing her mum or dad get hurt.

3. ***Who do you think is most likely to be responsible for Polly's injuries and why?***

   It could be either parent – or both, but the story suggests it is her mum. Traditionally, people expect it to be the man who is violent and aggressive but this is not always the case. A woman can abuse her male partner and her children.

   Whoever it is probably had a violent and abusive upbringing and so has learnt the behaviour from his or her own parents.

4. ***Is it possible or likely that anyone else in the family was at risk too?***

   If Polly has siblings then it is extremely likely that they would get similar treatment. The non-abusive parent may also get hurt.

5. *Suggest reasons why Polly tried to hide the fact that she was being abused.*

   - She'd been threatened that the family would be split up if anyone were to find out.
   - She'd been threatened that she would be hurt even more if she told.
   - She didn't want to upset the non-abusive parent (assuming there is one) because she'd been asked to promise to keep it a secret. This would be even more likely if it was her mum alone who abused her – it is proportionally rarer for a man to be abused by a female partner and is therefore more of a taboo subject.
   - She was frightened at what might happen. Although she wasn't happy at home, she didn't want to be put with strangers in a strange place. There was comfort in the life she knew – she felt more secure because it was familiar to her.
   - She was worried about what might happen to her non-abusive parent (assuming there is one) if she left – that parent might get seriously hurt or killed if she wasn't there to protect him or her.
   - She felt ashamed she had let this happen to her. She did not want friends and others to know that one of her parents thought so little of her that they regularly hurt her.
   - She may have felt that she was to blame for her parent's treatment of her – that she had, in some way, deserved it.

6. *Give as many examples as you can about ways in which a child can be abused.*

   - Physical (assault) or emotional mistreatment (mental abuse).
   - Sexual abuse. (Includes using the child for pornographic purposes or for prostitution.)
   - Neglect – neglecting the child's need to be loved or to be given the necessary stimulation for development, having poor nutrition, a lack of warmth and cleanliness, and a lack of suitable clothing.
   - Preventing a child from going to school or from receiving an education.
   - Abandonment.

- Not ensuring the child's safety. (For example, exposing the child to a risk of burning by not having a fireguard over a fire and not having a safety gate at the top of stairs to prevent a young child from falling down.)

- Giving alcoholic drinks or non-medicinal drugs to a child.

- Exposing the child to unnecessary risk or suffering. For example, not taking the child to a doctor when he or she is ill.

- Giving drugs to sedate or poison the child.

7. *What would you do if you were being abused? (If you really have been abused you may not wish to talk about it in front of others.) Is that the best way of dealing with the problem?*

(Personal responses required.)

8. *How would you feel if you were abused? Would you feel, in any way, that you deserved it?*

(Personal responses required.)

9. (a) *People can suffer years of abuse from their partner without seeking help. Why do abusers get away with it so often?*

Abusers get away with it because they have learnt how to manipulate people into being frightened of getting help. Once they have cut off the victim's social support, they gain more power. Many abusers discourage their partners from having regular contact with friends and make it difficult for them to invite friends to the home.

Abuse can happen in any relationship whether heterosexual or homosexual. Women or men can be abusive.

(b) *Why do their partners protect them?*

- Because they fear the humiliation of others finding out how they have been treated.

- Because their self-esteem is so low they cannot bear their problems being known about outside the house.

- Because the abuser often makes up and promises never to hurt them again. They probably like to believe this as it is the easiest course to take – and he or she may well love the abusive partner.

- Because it is easier to keep the status quo that exists. The victim needs great courage to leave an abusive household. It is a complete upheaval.

- Because they may not be able to face what might happen to them when their partner 'catches up with them'.

- Because the thought of a complete break, acting alone, may be too daunting. If the victim is a woman, for example, she may need to go to a women's refuge and 'hide' from her partner. It is not easy to start a new life when you feel low and lack confidence.

10. (a) *What do you think will happen to Polly's family in the longterm?*

- One (or both) parents might be prosecuted for abusing Polly.

- If only one parent is being abusive, he or she may be made to leave the family home by a court judgement.

- The children (if there are siblings) may be checked on at regular intervals by Social Services.

- Polly would be put on a Child Protection Register.

- Social Services may try to help the non-abusive parent care for Polly.

- Polly might be taken into care – and even adopted. Her parent(s) may lose their rights to have contact with her.

- Her siblings may be taken into care, even if there is no evidence of their being abused. It is enough that another sibling within the household has been mistreated.

- Her parents may split up. The non-abusive parent (if there is one) may have been given the necessary jolt by having it in the open to stand up to the abusive partner and leave with the children, or get a restraining order so that the abusive partner can no longer go to the home or be with the children.

(b) *How might the intervention change their lives?*

- Polly might need to be brought up in care. She might no longer feel afraid of being mistreated but she would probably miss her parents.

- Polly might be offered counselling.
- Polly might be put on a Child Protection Register and be checked on at regular intervals by Social Services.
- Polly might be split up from her brothers and sisters – they might be placed in different care homes or with different foster families.
- If the non-abusive parent (assuming there is one) were to start afresh with just the children, without his or her partner, the family would be able to stay together and Polly might have a happy home-life.

(c) Would Polly feel guilty about the part she had played in this?

Yes, she probably would, despite the fact that getting help is the right thing to have happened. She might feel her parents blame her for what has happened rather than recognising that they were responsible for their own actions and must take the consequences. Even if only one parent was abusive, the other allowed it to continue by not getting help.

STORY 19: I Don't Remember

The bouncers at the door frisked Richard and Mark before they went into the disco. They gave in their jackets, one part of a raffle ticket was taped to each and they were given the other halves so that there would be no mistake when they picked them up later.

After a casual look round the disco, which was well underway, Richard went to the men's toilets. They were empty. Mark stood guarding the door to the toilets in case someone came. Richard went into a cubicle, locked the door and climbed onto the toilet seat to open a small window at the top. Simon was outside and climbed onto the windowsill to hand Richard a bottle of whisky. Then he walked round to the entrance to be checked by the bouncers.

Throughout the evening the bottle of whisky changed hands and frequent visits were made to the toilet to drink from it. The bouncers hadn't spotted it this time.

The boys danced, ogled girls and drank. An occasional cigarette was lit.

At the end of the disco, the three of them left with the rest of the crowd. Another bottle of whisky waited for them by the big steel rubbish bins outside. They had hidden it earlier. Simon was staying the night at Richard's house but as Mark had to get home, they walked in the direction of his house. Richard's mum didn't wait up for him so he and Simon had plenty of time.

They swigged as they went and staggered and laughed. It was a great night.

As they passed the gates of the primary school, they decided to climb in. They wandered round the schoolyard and smashed the empty bottle against a wall, watching it scatter glass. Then they walked round the buildings, peering in and trying doors but they were locked. Mark stayed back to climb a wall.

Richard and Simon found themselves back at the gates and automatically scrambled back over and lurched their way to Richard's house.

Mrs Collins was woken early by a knock at the door. Her heart sank as she saw the blue uniform framed by the glass panel of the door, wondering what Richard had been up to this time. He was nothing but trouble.

The policeman explained his purpose and Mrs Collins led him upstairs to where Richard and Simon were sharing a room.

'I'm trying to trace the whereabouts of Mark Stanton. Mrs Stanton seems to think Mark was out with you last night. At a disco.' The policeman found it hard to breathe in the stuffy room. The smell was stomach-churning.

Richard rubbed his eyes. He felt sick and his head hurt. 'Yeah. He was.'

'Can you tell me where you last saw him?'

Richard thought but the last memory was of them leaving the disco together. Hadn't Mark gone straight home? 'I don't remember.'

'This is important, he's been reported missing. What about your friend? Was he with you too?'

Simon was just as confused as Richard. Hadn't Mark gone home after they'd split up? But Simon didn't even remember where they had split up.

The policeman sighed. 'Which way did you come home from the disco? Can you outline the route you took – in as much detail as possible?'

Richard's mind was a blank.

'Didn't we go most of the way with him?' Simon asked Richard.

'I think so…' Richard said doubtfully.

'Was Mark under the influence of alcohol too?' The policeman asked, as it was obvious that the boys had hangovers.

'Yes,' they admitted, avoiding Mrs Collins' eyes.

On Monday morning, the school caretaker came across Mark's body at the bottom of a wall. He had fallen off and banged his head. And he was dead.

Author's note: *This story is roughly based on an actual event where a young man had been unwittingly left to die by his friends who were too drunk to notice his absence.*

Discussion Sheet 19: I Don't Remember

1. What are the effects of drinking alcohol? Group them into positive and negative effects.

2. What are the signs of alcoholic drinking getting out of control on a daily basis (tending towards alcoholism)?

3. How were you brought up? Were you allowed alcohol from a young age or was it forbidden at home? Has this affected your approach to drinking now?

4. (a) The legal age limit for buying alcohol is 18. Have you succeeded in buying it under age?

   (b) Why is there an age-limit restriction?

5. Think of as many reasons as you can why there are bouncers at discos to check for weapons, illegal substances (drugs) and alcohol.

6. Should someone under the influence of drugs or alcohol be held responsible for his or her actions? Give reasons.

7. (a) In Britain, it is socially acceptable to drink alcohol. This is not the case in all cultures. Would you respect a teetotaller's wishes or would you be tempted to 'spike' his or her drink?

   (b) Can you think of a situation where it would be very dangerous indeed to spike someone's drink?

8. (a) What do girls think of boys who don't drink? How do boys regard other boys who don't drink? Britain is a macho society where men must be men to win approval – have you ever felt pressurised to drink alcohol so as not to feel left out?

   (b) How could you refuse alcohol without feeling stupid?

9. (a) Why do people smash beer bottles in the streets, car parks and children's schoolyards?

   (b) Have you ever done it yourself? If so, why?

10. (a) Do you use alcohol as an emotional prop? For example, some men might use alcohol to give them courage when asking a potential partner out.

   (b) What is use and what is abuse of alcohol?

Leader Sheet 19: I Don't Remember

1. *What are the effects of drinking alcohol? Group them into positive and negative effects.*

Positive:

- It reduces anxiety.
- It can make people feel more confident.
- It reduces inhibitions so that people are more relaxed and outgoing.
- It dilates the blood vessels so that the drinker feels warm.
- Small quantities of red wine have been suggested to have a positive affect on the heart.
- Drinking small quantities of alcohol in some cultures is considered sociable.

Negative:

- Reducing inhibitions can make people enjoy themselves more but it can also make them behave in a way that is uncharacteristic of them when they are sober. For example, someone might have sex when drunk, but regret it the following morning. A reduction of inhibitions also means that someone's conscience is dulled so that the person may commit a crime he or she normally wouldn't commit.
- A drunk person may be less able to control his or her emotions, becoming violent and angry or maudlin and weepy.
- Reaction times are slowed, judgement can be poor and control of body movement is impaired. This is very significant for those who drive or operate machinery under the influence of alcohol.
- Speech can become slurred.
- A drunk person can lose bladder and bowel control.
- A drunk person may feel sick and vomit.
- Death can occur from acute alcohol poisoning or from choking on vomit while unconscious.

- The person may not be able to remember what he or she did as alcohol can cause blackouts. (A sort of brief amnesia.)
- It can leave you with a hangover the following day.
- Alcohol can be addictive and the person may become dependent on it, becoming an alcoholic.
- Some medicinal drugs must not be mixed with alcohol as their combined affects are unsafe.
- Large quantities of alcohol reduces sex drive and contributes to infertility.
- In the longterm, the liver and brain may become damaged or cancers of the mouth and throat may develop. It can also cause gastritis, pancreatitis and duodenal disorders.
- It can raise blood pressure and increase the risk of having strokes.
- Heavy drinking over time can damage your brain (memory loss) and can change your personality.

2. *What are the signs of alcoholic drinking getting out of control on a daily basis (tending towards alcoholism)?*

- Finding empty bottles or cans of alcohol that the person has drunk alone.
- Always smelling alcohol on the person's breath.
- Finding the person drinking in secret.
- The person being unusually aggressive.
- The person having unsteady hands.
- The person needing to drink to perform everyday tasks.
- The person having bloodshot eyes.

3. *How were you brought up? Were you allowed alcohol from a young age or was it forbidden at home? Has this affected your approach to drinking now?*

(Personal responses required.)

4. *(a) The legal age limit for buying alcohol is 18. Have you succeeded in buying it under age?*

(Personal response required.)

(b) Why is there an age-limit restriction?

To protect young people from drinking in excess and damaging their bodies. It is also easier for young people to become addicted.

5. **Think of as many reasons as you can why there are bouncers at discos to check for weapons, illegal substances (drugs) and alcohol.**

   - To protect all the disco-goers.
   - To protect the people working at the disco.
   - To prevent the disco from being shut down in the event of negligence being proved.
   - To prevent violence.
   - To prevent drug dealing.
   - To prevent people vomiting all over the place.
   - To prevent the risk of collapse from adverse side effects.
   - To prevent any deaths from drugs or violence occurring on the premises.
   - To prevent vandalism.
   - To act responsibly.

6. **Should someone under the influence of drugs or alcohol be responsible for his or her actions? Give reasons.**

   Yes: Otherwise who is accountable for what happens? However, courts can look upon someone more leniently if the person was not aware of what he or she was doing. This does not mean that it is OK for offences to be repeated, using alcohol or drugs as a shield.

   No: It might be the person's first time getting drunk or trying out an illegal drug and they should not be blamed for effects that could not have been predicted by the person.

7. **(a) In Britain, it is socially acceptable to drink alcohol. This is not the case in all cultures. Would you respect a teetotaller's wishes or would you be tempted to 'spike' his or her drink?**

   (Personal response required.)

(b) Can you think of a situation where it would be very dangerous indeed to spike someone's drink?

If someone was on medication, it might be very dangerous to mix it with alcohol or an illegal drug. You might not necessarily know if the person was taking medication. Many drugs are taken regularly by people to keep certain conditions under control, for example, epilepsy drugs.

8. **(a) What do girls think of boys who don't drink? How do boys regard other boys who don't drink? Britain is a macho society where men must be men to win approval – have you ever felt pressurised to drink alcohol so as not to feel left out?**

    (Personal responses required.)

    (b) How could you refuse alcohol without feeling stupid?
    You could say:

'It's against my religion.'

'I can't. I'm driving.'

'I need to be clear-headed to do my homework.'

'Alcohol makes me ill.'

'I can't because of a medical condition (or because of my medication).'

'I can't because I'm training.'

'I don't want a drink. I'm fine as I am.'

'I don't like it, so I don't drink it.'

9. **(a) Why do people smash beer bottles in the streets, car parks and children's schoolyards?**

    * Because they think it's fun.
    * Because they feel anti-social and want to fight against authority and good behaviour.
    * Because they are thoughtless and do not think of the people who might get hurt or the people who have to clear up after them or the damage they might cause.

    (b) Have you ever done it yourself? If so, why?
    (Personal responses required.)

10. (a) Do you use alcohol as an emotional prop? For example, some men might use alcohol to give them courage when asking a potential partner out.

(Personal response required.)

(b) What is use and what is abuse of alcohol?

Use:

- Drinking socially when you are with others to enjoy the atmosphere and the warm feelings it gives.
- Drinking to celebrate a special occasion.

Abuse:

- Drinking with the sole purpose of getting drunk.
- Drinking to dull your feelings on a regular basis because you cannot cope with what is happening in your life.
- Drinking sufficient to make your behaviour offensive to others.
- It is an offence to drive or operate machinery, mechanical or electrical equipment with more than a certain amount of alcohol in the bloodstream. In some countries it is an offence to drive with *any* amount of alcohol in the bloodstream. In Britain, the maximum amount of alcoholic drink allowed while driving is four units*, but depending on your size or sex, even this may be sufficient to fail the breath test. (Women can be more affected than men drinking the same amount because their bodies hold less water and so the alcohol is more concentrated.)
- It is dangerous to drink alcohol before going swimming or taking part in other active sports.

* 1 unit = 1/2 pint beer or cider = 1 glass wine = 1 measure spirits

STORY 20: *Joyrider*

'My dad says I can have my own car as soon as I pass my test,' Terry boasted.

'I wish I had a dad who'd give me a car,' Ralph moaned. 'We've barely got a car as it is.'

'What do you mean?' Terry asked. Anything to do with cars interested him.

'There's always something going wrong with it. At the moment, the locks don't work. Mum doesn't think anyone would want to steal it but you can never be sure,' Ralph said, repeating his mother's words.

'Which area do you live in then?' Terry asked.

'Oh, by the repair garage.'

'Yeah, but which street?'

Ralph told him.

'Bit risky, there. What sort of car is it?'

'An Escort. No one would want to nick it, it's too old. The paint's peeling off down one side.'

Two days later, Melanie Cooper got her three-year-old ready and called up the stairs to her son. 'Ralph, it's time to go. If we leave it any later there'll be queues in the shops.'

She picked Rowena up and took her out to put her in the car seat. Melanie stood shocked. The drive was empty. Her legs felt weak and she thought she was going to be sick. Why did bad things keep happening to her?

Melanie went back inside with Rowena and took off her coat. She started to shake. She knew that she had to stay calm because of the children and cope with a phone call to the police. She'd had to cope with many things since her husband had been killed.

The police promised her car would turn up sooner or later. But without a car she could not claim on the insurance for some time – and not at all if they knew it hadn't been locked. Rowena couldn't walk far without a pushchair and it was in the boot. Useless.

Ralph thought it strange that he had only been saying the other day that he hoped it wouldn't be stolen and now it was. It made him feel superstitious.

Melanie had to ring her mum for help. She hated having to do it, as she liked to feel independent. She felt very angry with whoever had stolen her car. They had put her in this position.

The following day the police came with some 'good' news. They had found her car in the local woods. It had been used for racing and had crashed. Probably a write-off, so that would speed up the insurance for her. They arranged to have it towed home.

Melanie sighed in partial relief. At least she could get about now as the pushchair would be back and she could get taxis or ride in Mum's car safely using Rowena's car seat.

The car arrived that afternoon. She felt grief at seeing her means of greater freedom gone. Also, it had been the family car when John was still alive. Another part of that life ended.

Ralph examined the outside of the car closely. It would make a good story at school. Melanie opened the boot. Empty. She opened the front door. No car seat.

How could they have done this to her? She then looked at the front. No radio/cassette player. But worst of all, no tapes. She felt torn apart. That was the ultimate violation.

Melanie sat down on the seat and cried. And cried. The last reminder of John's voice had gone forever. The sound of John reading out bedtime stories to Ralph when he was younger was gone. And so was John. Forever.

Author's note: *The loss of a deceased's voice on tape is based on an event that actually happened under similar circumstances.*

Discussion Sheet 20: Joyrider

1. Why do you think Melanie's car was stolen?

2. Name the people who were affected in some way in the story and explain how they were affected.

3. How would it affect *you* if your family car (if you have one) was stolen and not replaced for three months?

4. Has the story changed any of your views on joyriding? If so, what were they and why?

5. Do you feel that joyriding is acceptable as long as the stolen car is a company car or from someone who can afford the loss?

6. Why do you think people joyride? Think of as many reasons as you can.

7. Some detention centres encourage joyride offenders to learn car maintenance and drive the cars they work on in the hope that they will not re-offend. This has been partially successful. Is there any way that teenagers can be somehow diverted from stealing cars in the first place?

8. Do you know of joyriders yourself or have you been involved in joyriding? If so, what was your reaction?

9. (a) Do you know the financial effect of someone filing a claim with their insurers? What happens to their premiums? Do they get fully reimbursed for the damage or loss?

   (b) If someone is maimed by a joyrider does he or she get compensation?

10. If you knew someone had killed or maimed a child joyriding would you tell the police, think it none of your business or be too scared to come forward? Give reasons.

Leader Sheet 20: Joyrider

---

1. *Why do you think Melanie's car was stolen?*

Ralph had told Terry about the car not locking – and Terry either stole the car himself (with friends) or told someone else about it.

2. *Name the people who were affected in some way in the story and explain how they were affected.*

> Melanie: She had lost her independence and now had to rely on her mum for help – something she didn't like doing.
>
> She had also lost her daughter's buggy and car seat, so she'd have to buy them again. The insurance money may pay for it but claimants don't always get enough to replace everything with new items.
>
> She'd have to buy another car, but finding one cheap enough to buy with the insurance money may mean it won't be so reliable. The last one had been theirs for years and they knew it well.
>
> She'd lose her no-claims bonus. (Unless it was protected by paying extra. But this is doubtful if she is financially challenged.) This would make the insurance for her car significantly greater. She may not be able to afford to replace it.
>
> She'd lost the sound of her husband's voice on tape.
>
> Ralph and Rowena: They'd lost the sound of their father's voice, which may have been precious to them. They were also inconvenienced by not having a car, and Rowena by not having a buggy.
>
> Melanie's mum: She'd been called upon to help out. She may do this willingly but it might not have been convenient for her.
>
> The police: Having to look for a stolen car means they cannot be following up other, more serious crimes.
>
> The insurers: Paying out on many claims raises the premiums for all.

3. *How would it affect you if your family car (if you have one) was stolen and not replaced for three months?*

(Personal response required.)

---

4. *Has the story changed any of your views on joyriding? If so, what were they and why?*

(Personal responses required.)

5. *Do you feel that joyriding is acceptable as long as the stolen car is a company car or from someone who can afford the loss?*

(Personal response required.)

6. *Why do you think people joyride? Think of as many reasons as you can.*

- They haven't passed their driving test because they can't afford to learn to drive, or are too young to learn. Or they may have had their licence taken away from them for dangerous driving.
- It is fun and 'cool'.
- They are speeding with other people's cars and so do not have to worry about the expense of repairs.
- They are bored with their lives and want to spice them up.
- They are with a group of friends who do it and don't have the bottle to say 'no'.

7. *Some detention centres encourage joyride offenders to learn car maintenance and drive the cars they work on in the hope that they will not re-offend. This has been partially successful. Is there any way that teenagers can be somehow diverted from stealing cars in the first place?*

- Have organised clubs or activities in the evenings to get teenagers off the streets.
- Try to ensure that, in school, each pupil is valued and involved in some way.
- Talk to teenagers to show the damage that can be done with joyriding – for example, giving the statistics of the numbers of joyriders and innocent people who get killed. Show how the loss of cars affects the victims. Show photographs or police videos of crashes.
- Give teenagers assertiveness training classes so that they learn to stand up for themselves and take responsibility for what they do.

- Identify possible future offenders early on – before they reach teenage years – and try to turn around the disaffected, the children who have started to show anti-social tendencies and tendencies to defy those in authority. This might be achieved through counselling or group work to help children deal with their personal problems so that they do not release their frustration in negative and damaging ways.

8. *Do you know of joyriders yourself or have you been involved in joyriding? If so, what was your reaction?*

(Personal response required.)

9. (a) *Do you know the financial effect of someone filing a claim with their insurers? What happens to their premiums? Do they get fully reimbursed for the damage or loss?*

- Claimants do not always get reimbursed for the full amount. For example, there is often £50 or £100 excess to pay – so the victim will have to pay the first part of the claim.

- The victim may also lose his or her no-claims bonus, making the next year's insurance more expensive.

- The victim may not get the full value of the car – its value would be independently assessed (assuming it is a 'write-off').

(b) *If someone is maimed by a joyrider does he or she get compensation?*

Someone who gets maimed by joyriders would not be insured, so no compensation would be given. Joyriders don't have insurance themselves and the person whose car it is may not be insured for all drivers – and even if he or she was, joyriders don't drive with the owner's permission. And joyriders often don't have a valid driving licence or haven't even passed their test.

10. *If you knew someone had killed or maimed a child joyriding would you tell the police, think it none of your business or be too scared to come forward? Give reasons.*

(Personal responses required.)

STORY 21: *I Never Have Any Nice Clothes*

'I've asked my mum for new trainers for Christmas,' declared Sharon as they were walking home from school.

'Me too,' Dara Childs told them. Hers were grimy and falling apart.

'Where from? The market?' Tracy taunted. 'That's where you get all your clothes isn't it? Good bargains are they?'

'No, I don't!' Dara denied hotly.

'You mean you sometimes go to Oxfam for a change?' Sharon laughed.

'I wouldn't be seen dead in your clothes. And you even let your mum cut your hair. No one's allowed to touch mine except the hairdresser!' Tracy boasted.

'Drop it, shall we? Dara's poor, isn't that right?' Sharon announced, embarrassing Dara even more before they split up to go home.

'Mum, I want Reebok trainers for Christmas. I don't want another pair from that market. They fall apart in no time. I tried Tracy's on as she's the same size as me and they were so much more comfortable,' Dara said as soon as she got in.

'But Dara, you know we can't afford fancy labels,' Mrs Childs explained.

'I never have any nice clothes. They're cheap and they look cheap. You want me to be the laughing stock of the school! You don't care!'

'Can you get any more overtime before Christmas, Eddie? Dara's desperate for Reebok trainers. I think her friends are giving her a hard time because they've got better clothes.' Mrs Childs looked worried.

'I've already told you, everyone's after overtime at the moment. Besides, I'm too tired to do any more. I did extra for her birthday but she's already outgrown the Levi's and that jumper's tight on her too. It's not worth it until she stops growing. And who says more expensive things are better?'

'Maybe I'll be able to do more then,' Alison mused.

'Look. Leave it. She'll understand the value of money even less if she gets everything she wants. She can wait until she's old enough to start earning herself.' Eddie was firm.

'But it's for Christmas, she'll be so disappointed!'

'I'm disappointed every day of my life but that doesn't mean I get someone showering me with expensive clothes. I'm not happy about it, but it's not something we can change. We just don't have the money for extras. I've made sure she's clothed, haven't I? Does she ever want for things to wear? No.'

'I know, but her friends at school have so much more and of better quality. It upsets her so.'

'Then she should change her friends!' Eddie stormed out of the room.

On Christmas day, there was only one parcel for Dara under the tree from her parents. She slowly unwrapped it, knowing it must contain new trainers but she hoped and hoped they'd be Reebok. Dara knew it would spoil her whole Christmas if they weren't.

Alison and Eddie Childs sat behind her, waiting for the moment, their arguments of weeks ago forgotten.

'Mum, Dad. Thank you!' There were tears in Dara's eyes as she went to kiss them.

Alison and Eddie looked at each other. It had been worth it. And chances were Dara would never notice that Great Grandma's crystal decanter was missing.

Discussion Sheet 21: I Never Have Any Nice Clothes

1. Does it matter what clothes and footwear you have? Why?

2. Were Sharon and Tracy good friends to Dara? Why?

3. Could Dara have said something to her friends to make the situation less painful for herself?

4. How would you react if someone criticised the quality or cost of your clothes?

5. Should Dara have asked her mother for Reebok trainers? Explain your reasons.

6. What are the pros and cons of having a school uniform?

7. (a) How must it feel for Dara coming from a family that has to count its pennies?

    (b) What must it be like for her parents?

8. How much understanding of Dara's circumstances did Sharon and Tracy show?

9. Why do you think Dara's father stormed out of the room when told about what Dara wanted? (Think of the role men are expected to play in Western society.)

10. Should children hide their disappointments from their parents and guardians? Give reasons.

Leader Sheet 21: I Never Have Any Nice Clothes

1. Does it matter what clothes and footwear you have? Why?

Yes:

- It is important to look your best – it helps you feel confident and have high self-esteem.
- You feel like the odd one out if you don't have the same sort of clothes as your friends.
- Young people need to be fashionable or they get laughed at.
- You could be bullied if you don't wear the right gear.
- You can't make a good impression on people if you don't look right.

No:

- What matters is the person you are and how you behave towards others. Clothes are an external, unimportant part of your life.
- It's a waste of money buying designer clothes. There are plenty of cheaper, alternative clothes around that are just as good quality but half the price.
- It shows a lack of individuality going with the crowd. It's as though you can't develop your own taste or be an individual.
- People should respect you for who you are, not for what you wear.
- Why waste hard-earned money on non-essentials when such a large proportion of the population are worried about getting enough food to keep them alive?

2. Were Sharon and Tracy good friends to Dara? Why?

No they weren't because they made her feel uncomfortable about her clothes. Their behaviour was bullying behaviour – they intimidated her and made her feel small because she wasn't a replica of themselves. They did not show her respect or show understanding of her family's circumstances. They shouldn't 'judge a book by its cover'. They should have valued Dara for her personal qualities, which come from within.

3. *Could Dara have said something to her friends to make the situation less painful for herself?*

- She could have told them that their attitude was not that of supportive, caring friends.
- She could have explained that her family couldn't afford Reebok trainers and that it was unkind of them to make her feel bad about it.
- She could have said she was proud of her parents, they had always been there for her and it didn't make them less important in her eyes because they struggled to make ends meet.
- She could tell them that she would choose her friends more carefully in future.

4. *How would you react if someone criticised the quality or cost of your clothes?*

(Personal response required.)

5. *Should Dara have asked her mother for Reebok trainers? Explain your reasons.*

Yes:

- Her mother needs to know that Dara is suffering because she hasn't got the 'right' footwear.
- As the Reebok trainers were so important to Dara, it was only fair for her mother to be told – otherwise her mother wouldn't know what Dara would appreciate most in the line of presents.
- It doesn't hurt to ask – Dara's mother can always say 'no'.

No:

- It was unfair to put pressure on her parents when Dara knew that they were short of money and doing their best for her.
- It made her parents feel like failures for not providing what their daughter wanted.
- It put pressure on her father to work overtime when he was already overtired with his current commitments.

- Buying designer trainers is a waste of money and Dara shouldn't have expected her parents to pay double (or even more) just for a label.

6. **What are the pros and cons of having a school uniform?**

For:

- All pupils look the same so there is less difference between the children from well-off families and those from financially challenged families.
- The pupils look smarter.
- There is less possibility of pupils wearing unsuitable, high-fashion clothing for school.
- It helps stop bullying because of the clothes people wear.
- Parents and guardians can keep other clothes for 'best'.
- It identifies the children as part of a group when they go away on trips – they are more easily spotted.

Against:

- Uniforms can be pricey – particularly as more than one shirt etc. is needed for when it needs to be washed. Also, these clothes have no use out of school and cannot be worn in the holidays – so parents and guardians would have to buy other clothes too.
- It can be a nuisance trying to get the uniform washed, dried and ironed in time, particularly if there is only one spare shirt etc., since the child might spill food down him or herself each day.
- Uniforms identify the school a child attends and leave him or her open to bullying – particularly if pupils of one school are hostile to pupils of another.

7. (a) **How must it feel for Dara coming from a family that has to count its pennies?**

- She might feel guilty about having to ask for things that she knows her parents can't afford.
- She might feel angry with her parents, blaming them for the teasing she gets at school because of the clothes she wears.
- She might feel ashamed of her parents because they are not well-off.

(b) What must it be like for her parents?

- They might feel sad that they cannot give their daughter what she wants.
- They might feel guilty that Dara is not as well dressed as her friends.
- They might feel like failures because they don't look as though they are doing well.

8. How much understanding of Dara's circumstances did Sharon and Tracy show?

None. They probably knew that Dara's parents couldn't afford Reebok trainers but they didn't care. They used Dara for entertainment by making fun of her and watching her squirm.

9. Why do you think Dara's father stormed out of the room when told about what Dara wanted? (Think of the role men are expected to play in Western society.)

Dara's father probably felt a failure – he was doing his best but that wasn't good enough. In traditional Western society, men are often expected to be the earners and they may feel it reflects on them if there is not enough money in the house for essentials (even though Reebok trainers are not essential).

He probably also felt angry with Dara because she didn't appreciate what she already had or his efforts to provide to the best of his ability. He felt she shouldn't expect more.

10. Should children hide their disappointments from their parents and guardians? Give reasons.

Yes:

- It's kinder to the parents.
- It's unreasonable to expect parents to do everything for them and get them everything they want. It is behaving in a spoilt way for children to keep telling parents what they want and that what they already have is not good enough.
- They need to understand that life is full of disappointments and need to get used to how it feels.

No:

- If they always hide their disappointments, parents will not get to know their children well and will not understand them so well.
- They won't be able to understand their needs or their moods.
- It is good for children to share their feelings with their parents – it helps them to bond, forming a close loving relationship.

STORY 22: *Shoplifter*

Story A

Rachel went into Mothercare and placed several baby items on the counter. 'I want my money back on these. The baby miscarried.'

'Do you have a receipt?' the till operator enquired.

Rachel shook her head. 'Vouchers are no good to me as I'm not going to have a baby and I don't know anyone who is now.'

The till operator consulted with her superior and finally they allowed Rachel to have the money in exchange for the goods. Rachel left with a triumphant grin. Now for a bit more shopping.

She decided to top up her make-up store at home and went into the chemist's to do this. It was a busy Saturday and no one noticed as she pocketed the lipstick and mascara. It was so easy! Why pay for it when you could get it for nothing?

Next, she went to Marks & Spencers. She picked up a petticoat, took it to the ladies and tore off the price tag. Then she went to customer services and told them it was a birthday present that hadn't fitted. They didn't want to give her cash but she stood her ground and the long queue was getting longer and people were impatient.

Finally, Rachel decided on some sweets in Woolworths. They had her favourites and even invited customers to pick their own! Which, of course, she did.

Before Rachel left the shop, she felt a hand on her shoulder. She dodged, surprising the store detective, and ran, but her arm was grabbed. She thought she was safe until she left the shop, that they couldn't catch you inside the store – but she'd been wrong.

Woolworths took down her details and later circulated them round the other major stores in the town. Although Rachel had used a different name, the store assistants did remember her description.

Story B

Bridget admired Carmen's new pencil case. It was metal with a loose bottom, hiding pencils underneath.

'I can get you one if you like,' Carmen told her. 'My sister's boyfriend works in the warehouse where they store these. He's only allowed so many, though, so don't tell anyone else.'

'No, I won't. Thanks Carmen.' Bridget did wonder if this was true but she decided not to think too deeply about it as she really wanted a pencil case like Carmen's. Especially as so much of her stuff had gone missing. It would save her having to buy more.

It was three weeks before Carmen brought Bridget the pencil case. 'Sorry it took so long – my sister only went there again on the weekend. Can I borrow your history book? I didn't have time to do the homework and it'll make it quicker if I can see what you've written.'

Bridget handed it over, knowing she couldn't refuse because of the pencil case.

But the next day, when the history homework was due to be handed in, Carmen was away. Bridget persuaded Miss O'Connor to open Carmen's locker so that she could look for her history book. Miss O'Connor stood next to her and watched her.

Moving Carmen's books, Bridget saw her pens and pencils that had gone missing. And the fancy compass her dad had bought her. Carmen had stolen them. But why? She hadn't needed them.

Bridget couldn't get them back while Miss O'Connor was watching and her history book wasn't there either. She decided to have it out with Carmen when she got back. But how could she explain she'd been through her locker without her permission?

Discussion Sheet 22: Shoplifter

1. How can Bridget explain to Carmen about having gone through her locker?

2. (a) Why do you think people shoplift?

   (b) If you've done it, why?

    (c) What are the consequences of shoplifting for the rest of the population?

3. What attracts you to shoplifting and what puts you off?

4. Do you think that prosecution notices in shops deter people from shoplifting?

5. (a) Carmen has a rare illness called kleptomania. What is it?

    (b) Many shoplifters claim to have this illness as an excuse for their behaviour. What excuse would you use, or would you accept responsibility for your actions?

6. (a) Should Bridget have accepted the pencil case since she suspected it might be stolen?

    (b) Have you ever knowingly accepted stolen goods?

7. (a) Have you ever been burgled?

    (b) If so, what did it feel like to know your possessions had been searched and items dear to you stolen?

8. Would you confront a friend if you knew he or she had stolen from you? Or would you hope that it would stop, or guard your possessions more carefully?

9. (a) How would your parents or guardians react to you stealing?

    (b) Is it right to supplement your pocket money by helping yourself to money from their purse or wallet?

    (c) If you explained that you felt you needed more money would they listen? Would you blame stealing on your parents or guardians because you felt you were forced into it through lack of money?

10. What crimes are committed by young people?

Leader Sheet 22: Shoplifter

---

1. ***How can Bridget explain to Carmen about having gone through her locker?***

   By telling the truth. She had every right to try to hand in her homework and had no malice in mind.

2. **(a) *Why do you think people shoplift?***

   - Because they get a 'kick' out of it. They enjoy the challenge and the risk involved makes it exciting.

   - Because they can't afford to buy things.

   - Because they've been dared to do it by their peers or have to do it to be included in the group or gang.

   - Because they have emotional problems – something has gone wrong in their life and they do not know how to handle it. Shoplifting is an expression of distress.

   - Because they are part of organised crime and they do it to make money for the group.

   - Because they make thieving a profession and shoplift instead of doing paid work.

   - Because they put something in their bag by mistake – they could have been distracted by children or worries.

   (b) *If you've done it, why?*

   (Personal response required.)

   (c) *What are the consequences of shoplifting for the rest of the population?*

   The prices of goods increase and sometimes jobs are lost in an effort to cut back on losses due to thefts. Although it is not fair that the innocent have to pay in this way for other people's crimes, businesses cannot operate at a loss. The money has to be recouped somehow. Businesses have to make profits in order to continue trading, to pay their rents, rates and salaries and to buy stock. Shoplifting is anti-social and perhaps shoplifters do not realise the consequences of their actions. Or they may think that their contribution to a company's loss is so small it is insignificant. But with all the shoplifting that goes on being taken into account, the losses can be huge.

3. **What attracts you to shoplifting and what puts you off?**

Attracts: Getting something you really want without having to pay for it.

Indulging yourself with little effort – you wouldn't have to save up your earnings from your Saturday job.

It wouldn't matter if you didn't like it after all as you wouldn't have lost out financially.

It would show your friends that you're brave and things like shoplifting don't faze you.

Puts you off: The risk of getting caught.

The reactions of your parents or guardians if they were to find out.

The fear of the police getting involved.

The possibility of getting a criminal record.

The shame you would feel.

4. **Do you think that prosecution notices in shops deter people from shoplifting?**

They might deter the more timid shoplifters, but for the determined ones, obviously not or there wouldn't be so much shoplifting going on. However, they do make the shoplifter aware of the consequences of getting caught – the person cannot claim ignorance of what may follow.

5. **(a) Carmen has a rare illness called kleptomania. What is it?**

This is a behavioural disorder where the person has an overwhelming desire to steal, without needing the object of that desire or even wanting to profit from it.

(b) Many shoplifters claim to have this illness as an excuse for their behaviour. What excuse would you use, or would you accept responsibility for your actions?

(Personal response required.)

6. **(a) Should Bridget have accepted the pencil case since she suspected it might be stolen?**

Yes: She wanted it and it was easier to take it without asking further questions. And she wouldn't have been able to restore it to the rightful owner. She would have caused more trouble for her friend had she tried. One pencil case does not cause the owner any great loss, it's a petty crime.

No: Legally this was wrong – there are no extenuating circumstances for accepting stolen goods.

(b) Have you ever knowingly accepted stolen goods?
(Personal response required.)

7. **(a) Have you ever been burgled?**
(Personal response required.)

(b) If so, what did it feel like to know your possessions had been searched and items dear to you stolen?

- Your area of comfort and refuge had been defiled and you felt as though your possessions had been sullied or dirtied.
- You felt angry that someone had broken into your home and stolen from you.
- You felt bereft that family heirlooms had been stolen – your last link with loved ones who had died.
- You felt scared that someone you didn't know had been poking around in your home and wondered if that person could know you personally or be watching you without your knowledge. Had he or she been watching your movements to know when to break into the property?
- You felt sad because many of the things were irreplaceable.
- You felt irritated because you had the trouble of having to find proof of value for each stolen item and wait for your claim to be processed before replacing your goods. And many of them could not be replaced exactly.

8. *Would you confront a friend if you knew he or she had stolen from you? Or would you hope that it would stop, or guard your possessions more carefully?*

   (Personal responses required.)

9. *(a) How would your parents or guardians react to you stealing?*

   (Personal response required.)

   (b) Is it right to supplement your pocket money by helping yourself to money from their purse or wallet?

   No: There is no right about stealing, for any reason.

   Yes: It's their fault for not giving you enough pocket money. All your friends have much more to spend than you and you only take small amounts.

   (c) If you explained that you felt you needed more money, would they listen? Would you blame stealing on your parents or guardians because you felt you were forced into it through lack of money?

   (Personal responses required.)

10. *What crimes are committed by young people?*

    - Bicycle and car thefts (for joyriding, selling of spare parts or for selling the car).
    - Burglary.
    - Football hooliganism.
    - Graffiti.
    - Personal assaults (mugging, beating up, sexual and racial assaults and sexual and racial harassment, rape).
    - Ram-raiding (usually with a stolen vehicle).
    - Shoplifting.
    - Vandalism.

STORY 23: *My Mum's Not Well*

'Do you want to come round to my house Saturday afternoon?' Preeti asked Sally and Malika.

'Don't your parents mind us always going there?' Malika asked. 'Sally, can't we visit you for a change?'

Sally's heart sank. She had known the question would crop up some time. 'My mum's not well – she doesn't want me to have friends round.'

'What's wrong with her?' Malika persisted. She hadn't fully trusted Sally since she had discovered that Sally had tried to keep Preeti's lost bracelet for herself.

'I'm not sure, but she gets upset by anyone coming to the house.'

'What do you mean?'

'I don't know. Please, I'm not allowed to talk about it.'

Malika and Preeti looked at each other and shrugged.

'My house, then,' Preeti stated, smiling.

Sally dawdled home and let herself in with her key. Her mum was looking out of the window for her. She closed the door of the porch behind her and carefully took off her shoes and stowed them neatly in the corner where all outdoor shoes were kept. They weren't allowed in the house.

Next, she unlocked and opened the front door, stepped on the mat and hung her school bag on a peg. Then she hung her coat. Her mum supervised her from the open door of the sitting room. Next, Sally took off all her clothes and dropped them into the laundry bag by the front door. She checked that she had closed the front door properly and looked at her mum who nodded to show she was satisfied.

Totally naked, Sally walked upstairs to the bathroom while her mother whisked away the laundry bag. She put on rubber gloves before she loaded the washing machine with Sally's dirty clothes. Then she squirted disinfectant into the bag and wiped it clean before washing the rubber gloves and hanging them on a special peg to dry. The laundry bag was returned to the hall for when her husband came home.

Sally stood in the bath waiting for her mum to come up and watch her shower. If her showers weren't supervised, she'd only have to start again until her mum was satisfied that she really was clean. It was the same every day. And her mum would always be exhausted from all the housework. After her shower was complete, her bath towels would be carried downstairs in a plastic bag to join her clothes in the washing machine, and the bath and shower screen would be washed and squirted with disinfectant. This process would then be repeated after her father had had his shower. Then her mother would shower and clean it all again. Life at home was one big cleaning treadmill for her mother – but for herself and her father, it was a nightmare.

Sally never did anything at home without thinking about it first. She wasn't allowed to help her mother do the housework, as her mum wouldn't be convinced it had been done properly. The terrible thing was, Sally was now finding people at school dirty and she tried to avoid touching anyone as she walked down the corridors. Surely she wouldn't become like Mum?

As soon as her mum came into the bathroom, Sally began to shower. Her mum nodded at her after she'd washed her hair and handed her the clean bath towel. Once her body was dry, Sally's mum clenched her fists, pursed her lips against her disgust and leant forward. She could now kiss her daughter hello.

Discussion Sheet 23: My Mum's Not Well

1. (a) Sally's mum is suffering from a mental illness called obsessive–compulsive disorder (OCD). Have you heard of this illness or do you know of anyone who suffers from it?

   (b) How does the disorder show itself?

2. (a) What other mental illnesses do you know about?

   (b) What things increase the risk of someone becoming mentally ill?

3. Do you know anyone suffering from a mental illness? If so, what is their problem?

4. (a) What is your attitude towards mental illness?

   (b) Where have you got this from?

5. If someone in your family was (or is) mentally ill, would you and your family keep it a secret? If so, why?

6. Why is a mental illness regarded as shameful, but a physical illness regarded with sympathy?

7. (a) How is Sally affected by her mother's illness?

   (b) Is it fair?

8. (a) If you had a parent or guardian with OCD, what would you do?

   (b) What do you think Sally should do?

9. Is there a clear dividing line between someone who is house-proud, wanting a clean and tidy home, and someone who has OCD?

10. How would you react to your best friend telling you he or she was receiving help from a psychiatrist or psychologist?

Leader Sheet 23: My Mum's Not Well

1. **(a) Sally's mum is suffering from a mental illness called obsessive–compulsive disorder (OCD). Have you heard of this illness or do you know of anyone who suffers from it?**

(Personal response required.)

(b) How does the disorder show itself?

An obsession is a recurrent thought, idea, impulse or image. With OCD, the recurrent thoughts can be to do with:

- contamination (as in Sally's mum's case)
- doubt (having to keep checking that doors have been locked, the cooker switched off, whether your hands have been washed 'properly'…)
- having hurt someone accidentally (by knocking them over, poisoning them)
- violence (such as thoughts of killing your own child).

OCD affects men and women equally, although more women have obsessions to do with cleaning. It can begin in childhood and gets progressively worse over time. If you live with someone who has a mental illness, you are more susceptible to one yourself. Mental illnesses caught early are easier to treat and cause less disruption to the lives of sufferers and their families.

2. **(a) What other mental illnesses do you know about?**

- alcohol dependence
- Alzheimer's disease
- anorexia nervosa
- bulimia nervosa
- compulsions such as gambling
- delirium
- dementia
- depression
- drug dependence

- phobias
- schizophrenia

(b) What things increase the risk of someone becoming mentally ill?

- A lack of friends.
- Being a victim of a crime.
- Bereavement.
- Divorce.
- Going through the menopause.
- In adults, the lack of a supportive partner in whom you can confide everyday things.
- Marital problems.
- Sexual problems.
- Stress.
- Surgery, such as amputation, hysterectomy, mastectomy.

Mental illness is often caused by a reaction to stress and emotional turmoil.

3. Do you know anyone suffering from a mental illness? If so, what is their problem?

(Personal responses required.)

4. (a) What is your attitude towards mental illness?

Attitudes can be those of rejection, fear, blame, ignoring the problem.

(b) Where have you got this from?

Parents or guardians, friends and the media.

5. If someone in your family was (or is) mentally ill, would you and your family keep it a secret? If so, why?

(Personal responses required.)

(Many people are ashamed of mental illness and hide the fact that they, or another member of their family, suffers from an illness of this kind.)

6. ***Why is a mental illness regarded as shameful, but a physical illness regarded with sympathy?***

   People can identify more easily with someone suffering from an infection or a broken bone. Sympathy is immediately forthcoming. But with a mental illness, much of the person's distress and suffering are hidden from view, so the reasons for the outward signs of the stress are not understood. We also fear what we don't understand. We associate mental illness with mental asylums and with people having to be locked away from society for their own safety and the safety of others.

7. (a) ***How is Sally affected by her mother's illness?***

   - Sally cannot have a normal childhood. She can't breeze in after school and slump in front of the television for a while or wander into the kitchen for a drink and snack.
   - Life at home is regimented by her mum.
   - Sally can't have friends round.
   - She has the stress of hiding what's going on at home from other people.
   - She probably has to lie a great deal to cover up.
   - Sally has started to think other people are dirty – if this were to continue, she'd probably get as bad as her mum.

   (b) ***Is it fair?***

   No, it's not fair on Sally. She is a child who is being forced to adapt her life to cope with her mum's problems and isn't being given any support to help her deal with how they affect her life. When one member of a household is in distress it affects the rest.

8. (a) ***If you had a parent or guardian with OCD, what would you do?***

   (Personal response required.)

   (b) ***What do you think Sally should do?***

   Sally should talk to her dad and convince him that their mum has to have help. It would be best for all of them. Her mum is a slave to her own fears and obsessions, and her dad has been made to fall in line with what she wants to keep her mind at ease. Neither parent should expect Sally to have to live with the situation for years – they are neglecting her needs as a child. Although it is difficult for people to accept they need help, when it affects several people's lives, it is the best thing to do.

9. Is there a clear dividing line between someone who is house-proud, wanting a clean and tidy home, and someone who has OCD?

There is no clear dividing line between a house-proud person and one who has just started to have OCD. However, if someone doesn't want to leave the house until it is very clean and tidy, it is an indication that things have got out of hand. The problem can then develop into more and more fussiness until it takes over the person's life and interferes with the functioning of the entire family.

10. How would you react to your best friend telling you he or she was receiving help from a psychiatrist or psychologist?

Ideally:

- Without making fun.
- Without telling everyone.
- With sympathy.
- By asking the person to explain the problems he or she has and offer to help support him or her.

STORY 24: *I'm a Person Too*

My name's Kate and I've got a problem with my mum. She nags at everything I do (and don't do). There's no pleasing her. I wear too much make-up, spend too long in the bath, spend too long on the phone, wear scruffy clothes, come home late, don't tidy my room, don't do my homework, bunk off school, watch too much telly. You name it, she moans about it. 'Where are you going?', 'When are you coming home?', 'What are you doing?', 'Why haven't you...?' Nag nag nag.

I'm Lorna. I'm an unpaid slave who does nothing but shopping, cooking, cleaning, washing... all day, every day. And I get no word of thanks or any help. I've tried to reason with Kate, pointing out what's fair, but she doesn't listen. I've had enough of being general dogsbody. I've lost my identity and I want it back. I've got my own life to run.

I'm going out and still haven't had my bath. She's been in there for ages and it's not fair. I bang angrily on the door. 'Mum. What are you doing? When are you coming out?'

'I'm having a bath and I'm reading this really good magazine I bought. I'll come out when I'm ready.'

'You're making me late. You'll have to give me a lift.'

'No.'

'You've GOT to! I'll be late!'

'No. Now go away, you're disturbing my reading.'

My mum's going mad!

I felt so good after my bath that I cooked a special meal. I quite fancied eating on my own for a change for peace and quiet.

'Mum, what are you doing?'

'Loading the tray with my meal. Help yourself, it's ready whenever you want it. I'm going to eat in my room.' I lifted up the tray, balancing the bottle of wine carefully as it was very heavy. Kate just stood gawping.

Mum's been strange – she must have gone straight to bed after tea as she didn't even do the washing up. I hope she's better tomorrow, my clothes need washing.

I got up early to wash up the pots. I half hoped they'd have been done but I'd had a really relaxing evening and so didn't feel bad about doing them. Then I sat down in the sitting room with my coffee and toast.

'Mum! Look at the time! Why didn't you wake me? You can make me some toast but it had better be quick. I'll be late for school.'

'No.'

'What?'

'No. I don't want to.'

Kate stomped out of the room saying she wasn't hungry anyway and once she'd got her shoes and coat on slammed the front door. I went upstairs to sort the washing, which was strewn all over the floor of my bedroom, the bathroom and the landing. I put a load on.

'Where's my washing?' I asked Mum when I got home. It was all hers on the line.

'In your room.'

I went upstairs to look, not knowing what to make of her and couldn't believe my eyes. She'd thrown all my dirty laundry in my room.

'Mum! It's dirty! You haven't washed it! And you just threw it in!' I was very indignant. It wasn't fair. Other people's mum's didn't behave like this. 'When are you going to do it?'

'I'm not. I don't want to. Do you like my hair?'

I hadn't noticed she'd had it cut and styled until she patted her head. I ignored it.

'You'll have to do my washing tonight if it's going to be ready to iron tomorrow – I need it for Saturday night.'

'Kate, the washing machine is over there. It's quite simple to use. I'll see you later.'

'Are you going out?' I shouted and stamped my foot.

'Yes.'

'Where to? When will you be back?'

'I'm going for a drink and a meal. I'll be back when I'm ready. 'Bye!'

'What's for tea?'

'Whatever you find.'

Mum closed the front door behind her. She's gone mad. Utterly utterly mad. She's so irresponsible! I sat down bemused and thought about what to do.

When I got home, I noticed that the airer was full of Kate's clothes. The kitchen had a nasty burnt smell. I opened the window.

The next morning I thought I must have overslept as I heard Kate in the kitchen. I quickly pulled on my dressing gown and went downstairs.

'Would you like some coffee?'

I smiled. A really warm smile. 'Thanks. That would be lovely.' I took a sip of the hot brew and leaned back in my chair. It promised to be a good day.

'If you do my ironing, Mum, I'll clean the bathroom for you.'

We looked at each other across the table. Our eyes met. I was a person at last.

Discussion Sheet 24: I'm a Person Too

1. (a) Do your parents or guardians have rights?

   (b) Do they make them known to you and do they make sure that they are kept to?

2. List the rights you think your parents or guardians should have (with respect to you).

3. What are the rights you think you should have (with respect to your parents or guardians)? (Be sensible, honest and FAIR.)

4. Are your parents' or guardians' rights the same as those you want for yourself? (For example, the right to be free from fear or threat of violence.)

5. How do you treat your parents or guardians?

6. How do they treat you?

7. (a) What do you want changed?

(b) What is the fairest way to do it?

8. What methods have you already tried? Did any fail? If so, why do you think they failed? Can you think of any better ways?

9. What do your parents or guardians want changed? How would you like them to go about it?

10. (a) Explain as fully as you can the messages that the story was putting across.

(b) Did you learn from the story? If your parents or guardians were to read it, would they learn anything? If so, what?

Leader Sheet 24: I'm a Person Too

1. **(a) Do your parents or guardians have rights?**

   Yes, everyone has rights.

   (b) Do they make them known to you and do they make sure that they are kept to?

   (Personal responses required.)

2. **List the rights you think your parents or guardians should have (with respect to you).**

   They should have rights to:

   - privacy (such as not having their papers and bank statements gone through)
   - time alone
   - respect
   - consideration
   - not being embarrassed by you in front of friends
   - their property (such as not having something borrowed without their permission or not being stolen from)
   - not being woken up in the middle of the night by your phone calls
   - not being kept up worrying by your coming home late
   - expect you to take responsibility in the home by sharing chores
   - expect you to do your homework without having to be nagged
   - expect communal areas to be kept free from your mess
   - be free of fear or threat from you
   - your abiding by reasonable house rules and lifestyle rules
   - your not becoming involved in criminal activities
   - your not involving them with violent acts
   - not being expected to lie for you.

3. *What are the rights you think you should have (with respect to your parents or guardians)? (Be sensible, honest and FAIR.)*

You should have rights to:

- playing your music at reasonable hours
- being out until a reasonable time
- being free from fear or threats of violence
- food and warmth, and decent clothing
- not being embarrassed by your parents or guardians in front of your friends
- not having to do too many chores (some parents and guardians expect their children to take on all the housework as soon as they are able)
- privacy (such as not having your diary read or your things gone through)
- your property (such as not having something borrowed without permission or not being stolen from)
- respect
- time alone.

4. *Are your parents' or guardians' rights the same as those you want for yourself? (For example, the right to be free from fear or threat of violence.)*

Many of the rights are the same (as in the above suggestions).

5. *How do you treat your parents or guardians?*

(Personal response required.)

6. *How do they treat you?*

(Personal response required.)

7. *(a) What do you want changed?*

(Personal response required.)

(b) What is the fairest way to do it?

- By talking to your parents or guardians.

- By understanding there might be conditions attached.
- By being prepared to compromise.
- By also listening to their needs and taking them into account.

8. *What methods have you already tried? Did any fail? If so, why do you think they failed? Can you think of any better ways?*

(Personal responses required.)

9. *What do your parents or guardians want changed? How would you like them to go about it?*

(Personal responses required.)

10. (a) *Explain as fully as you can the messages that the story was putting across.*

- If you behave selfishly, you affect the lives of other people.
- If you want to be treated with consideration by your parents or guardians, you need to treat them with consideration.
- If you want favours done for you, you have to carry your share of the weight at times and offer to do favours for your parents or guardians in return.
- If you want to be treated with respect by your parents or guardians, you need to treat them with respect.
- Relationships are not one-way streets. Both sides have to work hard at them and one person cannot be benefiting all the time at the expense of another without resentment and arguments.
- You need to recognise that your parents or guardians have needs just like you.

(b) *Did you learn from the story? If your parents or guardians were to read it, would they learn anything? If so, what?*

(Personal responses required.)

Section 3

Introduction

Section 3 is concerned with issues relevant to 14- to 17-year-olds. Stories 31 and 32 are interconnected with a developing theme and should be read in order. The rest of the stories in Section 3 can be read in any order. Some of the characters in this section also appear in Section 4.

Section 3 largely concentrates on health, sexuality and sexual health.

Summary of Contents

Story	Title	Subject
25	No Thanks, I'm Not Hungry	Eating disorders
26	I'm So Tired	ME/chronic fatigue syndrome and depression
27	Hands Off!	Sexism, sexual harassment
28	He Was My Boyfriend!	Relationships
29	SIDA	AIDS
30	2052 AD	Smoking
31	The Party*	Pregnancy
32	Tina's Decision*	Pregnancy termination
33	No!!	Date rape; rape
34	TO LEAD BAGGY?	Homosexuality, homophobia
35	Perspective	Outlook on life

* Titles in succession are interconnected and should be read in order.

STORY 25: *No Thanks, I'm Not Hungry*

'No breakfast?' Maria Martinez asked her daughter, Elena.

'No thanks, I'm not hungry. I've got to go. I'm late.'

'Take some toast with you,' Mrs Martinez insisted while quickly wrapping it up.

'I told you…' Elena began heatedly and then broke off, sighing. It would be easier to just take the toast and go. 'Yes. Thanks Mum. 'Bye.'

'Don't be late and don't forget you still have some homework to do.'

'How could I with you to remind me?' Elena muttered as she left. It was only a short walk to the bus stop and as Elena approached Katya she dropped the toast into the litter bin.

'What was that?' Katya asked.

'Oh, the rest of my breakfast. Mum had made too much. Look, here's the bus. Shops here we come!'

Two hours later, Katya suggested they had a McDonald's.

'You can, but I'm not hungry. I'm still reeling from my breakfast,' Elena replied.

Katya frowned. When was the last time she'd seen her friend eat? At school, Elena claimed to have already eaten her lunch by the time Katya got to her – but it was more likely she'd lied about having it. 'Since when don't you like McDonald's?' she asked suspiciously.

Elena shrugged. 'I'm on a diet. I'm fat.'

Katya laughed. 'You're not. You're thinner than me! And anyway, your body shape changes when you're in your late teens. You lose any puppy fat if you've got it.'

'I'm not going to wait that long.' Suddenly, Elena looked round for a bench to sit on. She felt faint.

'What's wrong?' Katya asked in alarm as she noticed Elena had gone a sickly white colour underneath her olive skin.

After Elena had sat down, Katya demanded angrily, 'Exactly how much breakfast have you had? And what about all those lunches you said you'd eaten? No wonder you feel ill.'

'I'm fine,' Elena protested. 'It's just the time of the month.'

Katya looked disgusted. 'You said that last week to Ms Ahmed when you had to leave assembly because of feeling faint. And I can't believe you've got another period only a week later.'

'You're just jealous because I'll be thin and you won't,' Elena snapped back and stormed off, leaving Katya staring after her.

'You wanted to see me, Miss,' Elena stated as she entered her form room in the lunch hour later that week.

'Yes. Sit down.' Ms Ahmed waited until Elena was settled. 'Katya's told me you're crash dieting to the extent of missing meals altogether.'

Elena felt defensive. 'She's exaggerating. It's not like that.'

'What is it like then?' Ms Ahmed waited but Elena didn't reply. 'What did you have for lunch today, Elena?'

After a pause, Elena replied, 'An apple.'

'A whole apple?'

Elena shook her head. 'It was a very big apple.'

'I'm worried you're becoming anorexic,' Ms Ahmed told her gently, 'and I want to discuss it with your parents. You aren't fat and you'll make yourself ill if you stop eating.'

'I am eating. It's under control,' Elena said, defending herself.

'Do you make yourself sick or take laxatives?'

'No.'

'Good. Any pressures at home or school?'

Elena shook her head.

'Well, you're very bright so I can't see you struggling with your work. Or are you finding last year's grades hard to live up to?' Elena didn't reply. 'And your parents? They must be very proud of you and love you very much.'

'They don't love me!' Elena cried. 'Only my grades and homework. That's all they care about.' Elena burst into tears.

'I'm sure you're wrong.' Ms Ahmed wondered if Elena's starvation diet was a cry for help and understanding or self-punishment because she thought she was unloved and had low self-esteem. 'Do you have too much to live up to in terms of your parents' expectations?'

Elena lifted her eyes in misery. 'I don't know,' she whispered.

'Elena, we have to speak to your parents about this, to help you. You'll be seriously ill if this carries on.'

Discussion Sheet 25: No Thanks, I'm Not Hungry

1. Why was Elena dieting?

2. Under what circumstances would you, or do you, diet?

3. (a) What are the symptoms of anorexia?

   (b) Would you describe Elena as anorexic? Give reasons.

4. (a) Why is it not a good idea for young teenagers and children to diet without good reason and the support of a doctor?

   (b) What are the consequences of starvation?

5. (a) Do you know general characteristics of anorexics and their families?

   (b) What backgrounds make this disease more likely?

6. (a) Female anorexics outnumber males by more than nine to one. Why do you think that is?

   (b) Does the media encourage anorexia in its portrayal of 'attractive' men and women?

   (c) Are you influenced by the media?

   (d) Why do shops not display big-figured mannequins?

7. (a) Bulimia is an eating disorder that can be present at the same time as anorexia. What is it?

   (b) How does being bulimic affect the person's body?

8. What are the differences between bulimics and anorexics?

9. Do you change your intake of food under pressure, either by bingeing (eating much more) or by eating much less than normal? Do you ever eat food for comfort? Do you feel guilty if you have 'binged'?

10. Was Katya right to go to the form teacher about her worries over Elena or should she have taken some other action or ignored her friend's problem?

Leader Sheet 25: No Thanks, I'm Not Hungry

1. *Why was Elena dieting?*

To make herself thin because she didn't like herself as she was. She perceived herself as fat and unattractive and didn't feel that she was loveable as she was.

2. *Under what circumstances would you, or do you, diet?*

(Personal response required.)

3. (a) *What are the symptoms of anorexia?*

- A fear of fatness.
- Under-eating.
- Excessive weight-loss from not eating.
- Loss of periods (in girls).
- Initially sufferers are restless and hyperactive but as the illness progresses the sufferer becomes tired and weak.

Although anorexia means 'loss of appetite', sufferers do not lose their desire to eat but manage to control what they eat.

(b) *Would you describe Elena as anorexic? Give reasons.*

Yes: She is denying herself the food she previously enjoyed (such as the McDonald's) and is lying to cover up the fact that she has stopped eating. Also, her not eating is making her ill – she has twice nearly fainted. She also views herself as fat and unattractive which her friend and teacher do not agree with, so she probably has a distorted image of herself.

No: She doesn't sound as though she has had the symptoms of anorexia all that long and she has not been given an official diagnosis. It is dangerous to label people too hastily.

4. (a) *Why is it not a good idea for young teenagers and children to diet without good reason and the support of a doctor?*

- Because dieting can trigger anorexia, it is not sensible for people to diet unless they really need to – and a doctor is probably the best judge of that, certainly for young people where the risk of developing anorexia is so high. (About a third of anorexics are overweight when they start dieting but are then unable to stop once they have reached a desirable weight.)

- Young children and teenagers need food to grow and because they burn up so much energy (they tend to be very active). If they interfere with their diet without the guidance of a doctor they can have deficits in certain vitamins or minerals. For example, a person who avoids dairy products because they are fattening loses out on essential calcium. Teenagers' teeth can fall out and they can have brittle (easily broken) bones if they fail to have a balanced diet.

(b) What are the consequences of starvation?

- Abdominal pain.
- Becoming very sensitive to the cold.
- Brittle bones and weak teeth.
- Broken sleep.
- Depression.
- Difficulty in concentrating.
- Dizziness.
- Getting dry, discoloured skin.
- Growing downy hair all over the body.
- Losing hair from the head.
- Muscles becoming weak.
- Suffering severe constipation.
- Swelling, especially of the stomach, face and ankles.

If starvation continues, it can eventually lead to death. (Eating disorders have one of the highest mortality rates of all psychiatric illnesses. Over 10 per cent of sufferers die either from the effects of starvation or from committing suicide.)

5. (a) Do you know general characteristics of anorexics and their families?

Anorexics are often:

- anxious to please
- conscientious

- from tight-knit families
- highly intelligent
- introverted
- well behaved.

They can feel they are only loved for their achievements and may see dieting as a way of being in control of their own lives, especially if they have parents or guardians with great expectations. There is a higher incidence of anorexia in private schools than in state schools. It also seems that anorexics do not wish to grow up, wanting to keep their childhood shapes and excessive slimming helps this.

(b) What backgrounds make this disease more likely?

- One in 200 girls suffer from anorexia between the ages of 16 and 18 when the illness is at its peak. But sufferers can range from age 6 to 60.
- For ballet dancers, models and athletes the incidence rises to 1 in 20. (Great emphasis is put on body size and weight.)
- For middle-class teenage girls and young women, the rate is 1 in 100. (Family expectations are higher.)
- Girls in private schools are more than 5 times as likely (1 in 100) to suffer from anorexia than girls in a London comprehensive (1 in 550).

Anorexia is more prevalent in rich societies, in upper- and middle-class families and in those that go on to further education. (Statistics from The Eating Disorders Association.)

6. (a) Female anorexics outnumber males by more than nine to one. Why do you think that is?

- Because women may believe that to be accepted and admired by men they must look a certain way. Men may believe they have to be high achievers in life and have outgoing personalities to be attractive to women so are not so concerned about their appearance.
- Because men tend to use other outlets for their stress – drinking, smoking, doing sport or working out and becoming workaholics. Women are more likely to diet.

- Because women are inundated with details of diets and slimming foods in the magazines they read.
- Because women may fear their femininity and their possible failure as an adult woman. (Anorexic women heavily depend on others for approval.)
- Because some women are unhappy being female, believing that men have more opportunities and are more valued by society.

(b) Does the media encourage anorexia in its portrayal of 'attractive' men and women?

Models, whether male or female, do predominantly have slim and attractive bodies. In societies that do not value slimness, anorexia is rare. In environments that do value slimness such as in ballet, the incidence of anorexia is higher.

(c) Are you influenced by the media?

(Personal response required.)

(d) Why do shops not display big-figured mannequins?

Because the fashion industry believes its clothes will sell better on slim models, and have not manufactured large mannequins. It has been estimated that nearly 50 per cent of British women are a size 16 (UK) and over.

7. (a) Bulimia is an eating disorder that can be present at the same time as anorexia. What is it?

Bulimia involves binge eating (eating enormous amounts of food in a short space of time) and then taking steps to keep body weight down.

- Bulimics vomit so that the food does not have time to be absorbed by their bodies.
- Bulimics take laxatives as the eaten food moves faster through their gut and so there is less time for their body to absorb the food.
- Diuretics are used to expel water from their bodies, which also keeps their weight down.

(b) How does being bulimic affect the person's body?

Bingeing and then vomiting:

- Bingeing and vomiting can occur several times a day and in severe cases there is dehydration.
- Death can occur if the right mineral balance is not maintained for the body's organs to work. (Heart failure can result.)
- Epileptic fits can occur.
- Kidney damage can occur.
- Stomach acid from vomiting may damage the bulimic's teeth.
- The sufferer can have a puffy face from swollen salivary glands.

Using laxatives:

- Laxatives can give persistent abdominal pain.
- They may damage the bowel muscles leading to long-term constipation.
- They can also make fingers swell.

Using diuretics:

- Causes chemical imbalances in the blood, most commonly low potassium levels.
- Some diuretics can raise the amount of uric acid in the blood, increasing the risk of gout.
- Some diuretics increase the blood sugar level that can cause or make diabetes mellitus (a lack of insulin production) worse.

Bulimics also suffer from depression and may become suicidal.

8. *What are the differences between bulimics and anorexics?*

- Bulimics tend to keep their weight the same despite the huge quantities of food they consume. Anorexics, and anorexics who are also bulimic, continue to have a very low weight.
- Most bulimics are women between the ages of 15 and 30. Anorexia peaks in the teens.
- Bulimia is rarely found in men. (More so than with anorexia.) Women who suffer from pre-menstrual tension may be inclined to binge because their blood sugar level drops.

Many bulimic women lead successful and high-powered lives, using their bulimia as an outlet for stress and pressure.

9. *Do you change your intake of food under pressure, either by bingeing (eating much more) or by eating much less than normal? Do you ever eat food for comfort? Do you feel guilty if you have 'binged'?*

(Personal responses required.)

10. *Was Katya right to go to the form teacher about her worries over Elena or should she have taken some other action or ignored her friend's problem?*

She could have gone to Elena's parents – but they might be part of the problem. By going to a trusted teacher, Katya has ensured there is an outside party involved who could act as intermediary. Also, the teacher can guide the parents into seeking professional help for their daughter. With mental illnesses, some parents and guardians feel they need to cover up problems to save face.

Had Katya ignored Elena's problem it would be likely to get worse, and the longer anorexia goes untreated, like other mental illnesses, the harder it is to treat. She would be doing her friend a disservice if she did not get help for her, even though it was without her permission.

Author's note: A new food disorder called orthorexia (an as-yet unofficial term at the time of writing) is an obsessional interest in healthy eating where the sufferer can lose perspective, ruling out non-organic, frozen, high-fat, sugar- and salt-containing foods, and may eat only raw and natural produce. Consequently, he or she may become as thin as an anorexic and be missing vital nutrients. The orthorexic person can spend all his or her day thinking about, planning and preparing food.

STORY 26: *I'm So Tired*

Tim stared uncaringly out of the sitting room window on to the street. Another day ahead. Another day exactly the same as the day before and the day before that. In fact, he was likely to have the same day for a long time to come. Who knew when it would change?

Tim's head rested on the chair back and a padded footstool supported his feet. He'd never known anyone could be so tired for so long, without a break. He'd only eaten breakfast, washed and got dressed, and he felt worse than if he'd had a full day in school and partying on a Friday night.

His glandular fever had been bad enough. Because the tiredness had crept upon him so gradually, he'd thought he was only run down. Vitamins and early nights were what he'd needed. But the walk to school had become more and more like climbing a steep mountain. And when he'd arrived, he'd had to sit down with his head in his hands. The headaches had worried him but it wasn't until he kept feeling prickly hot for no reason and his throat became dreadfully sore that he told his mum. She took him to the doctor who took a swab from the back of his throat and blood from his arm. He was too tired even to think of leaving the house while he waited for the test result.

Even then, he hadn't understood what was wrong with him. He'd heard of glandular fever, other teenagers had had it and it was something to be dreaded but he hadn't understood why until then. His friends weren't allowed to visit. Their parents were too worried that they'd catch it. He felt as though someone had marked a cross on his door like they did in the days of the plague. He had chatted to them over the phone but it soon became obvious that their worlds were moving apart. He hadn't anything to say and his friends were coping fine without him. Even his best friend Jack had deserted him, becoming more friendly with the others.

Tim had heard that the others who had had glandular fever were back to normal in half the time he was. He'd had three months off school. But then he'd realised he hadn't got back to normal at all. Yes, he'd made it back to school feeling quite a lot better, but each day that followed was harder to cope with. He couldn't wait to get to bed after his evening meal and could not do his homework.

Tim recalled his last day in school. He'd felt dizzy and ready to throw up after he'd got there. And then he'd got to go to assembly. There'd been a bottle-neck in the corridor and there was a crowd of them waiting to get out of the classroom. Tim had felt weak and strange and suddenly he was on the floor. When they'd tried to get him up he couldn't move. He was too tired to do anything.

That had been seven months ago. Tim wondered what his friends were doing now. They had visited at first, when they were told he wasn't infectious, that the glandular fever was long gone. But gradually they stopped coming alto-gether. They were embarrassed about being with him. There were too many awkward silences. As soon as they started to talk about parties and discos, their voices trailed away, realising they'd been tactless. Jack had a girlfriend now and was always with her. Tim's mum had seen them together at the shops and she'd told him that Jack had pretended not to see her. He'd known she'd ask him why he hadn't visited her son lately.

Tim closed his eyes, exhausted by the morning's efforts. What was the point in life if all he had to look forward to was Mum looking after him like a baby or a sick old man? His life had hardly started but he felt as though it were at an end. He could cope so much better if only he didn't feel so bloody alone. No one understood. And only Mum cared, but it was too much for her on top of every-thing else she'd got to do. And he didn't want to be dependent on Mum – he wanted his own life back.

Discussion Sheet 26: I'm So Tired

1. The main theme of this story is ME or CFS (chronic fatigue syndrome). Sometimes it is called post-viral fatigue syndrome. What is it?

2. What are the symptoms of ME/CFS?

3. (a) What is glandular fever?

   (b) What are the differences between ME/CFS and glandular fever?

4. Have you had ME/CFS or do you know anyone with ME/CFS?

5. What sort of help do you think someone with ME/CFS who was able to attend school would need from the school?

6. If your friend had ME/CFS what could you do to help?

7. Tim is not very happy. Why is this?

8. What does it mean to feel socially isolated?

9. (a) Many chronically sick people suffer from depression. What is this?

   (b) Other people suffer from depression too. Can you give some examples?

10. What can be done to help a depressed person?

Leader Sheet 26: I'm So Tired

1. ***The main theme of this story is ME or CFS (chronic fatigue syndrome). Sometimes it is called post-viral fatigue syndrome. What is it?***

   (ME stands for myalgic encephalomyelitis.)

   ME/CFS is an illness that has many symptoms but the most apparent, and the one that characterises it, is extreme tiredness or exhaustion. The tiredness is far more severe than the tiredness people feel at the end of a busy day.

   Young people suffering from ME/CFS can be totally unable to care for themselves. Some, however, are able to attend school if they have considerable help.

   Often, it is triggered by a viral illness but in many people the exact cause is not known. Diagnosis is given after all other explanations have been ruled out.

2. ***What are the symptoms of ME/CFS?***

   (Not all symptoms have to be present for a positive diagnosis.)

   - Cold extremities.
   - Drug sensitivities.
   - Extreme fatigue (always present).
   - Fainting and feeling faint.
   - Headaches.
   - Insomnia.
   - Light intolerance.
   - Muscular pain.
   - Nausea.
   - Poor short-term memory.
   - Poor temperature control.

3. ***(a) What is glandular fever?***

   It is a viral illness with an incubation period of up to six weeks before symptoms of a sore throat, lethargy, poor appetite, fever, headache and swollen glands appear. These symptoms can last up to two weeks but the person may not feel well until several weeks or even months later, feeling tired and depressed. (Some people have glandular fever without realising it.)

(b) What are the differences between ME/CFS and glandular fever?

- Glandular fever is an infection due to the Epstein-Barr virus and is transmitted through saliva. There is no single cause for ME/CFS and it is not infectious. It often develops following an infection where the person has not fully recovered, but this is not so in all cases.

- Glandular fever occurs in adolescents and young adults, its incidence peaking between ages 15 and 17. ME/CFS peaks in adults at age 30 to 40 (although many children and younger adults do get it).

- The symptoms of glandular fever are not as severe or as long lasting as those of ME/CFS. It can take people a long time to recover from glandular fever, having post-viral fatigue, but this often improves over a period of several months. For ME/CFS to be diagnosed the person needs to have had the symptoms for at least six months and to have had his or her energy levels reduced by at least 50 per cent.

4. Have you had ME/CFS or do you know anyone with ME/CFS?

(Personal response required.)

5. What sort of help do you think someone with ME/CFS who was able to attend school would need from the school?

The school may need to:

- allow the person to attend on a part-time basis
- arrange for the person to have lifts to and from school
- excuse the person from games lessons
- understand the person's needs and understand that these may vary from day to day and week to week. People suffering from ME/CFS do not have consistent energy levels – they often have good and bad days
- inform all the teachers about the person's needs
- be flexible about deadlines

- be patient with the person and recognise when that person's limits are being pushed too hard
- provide a rest area so that the person can lie down if necessary
- be understanding about repeated absences and part-day attendance
- have certain lessons timetabled on the ground floor if the stairs are too much for the person to cope with.

6. *If your friend had ME/CFS what could you do to help?*
   - Help him or her to remember commitments.
   - Offer to carry his or her school bag.
   - Offer to fetch things that he or she needs.
   - Be understanding.
   - Be a good friend and understand if he or she is too tired to talk, but don't let the person become socially isolated. Be near.

7. *Tim is not very happy. Why is this?*
   - He is lonely – he spends all day everyday at home with his mother. He needs friends of his own age.
   - He is frustrated that he is physically unable to do much each day and sees his life wasting away before him, all his dreams and hopes for himself and his future melting away.
   - He feels unwell. It makes him feel vulnerable. No one feels happy or able to face hardships in life if they are feeling bad – and for so long. Problems are harder to cope with and have more impact than they would on someone who was feeling mentally very positive.
   - He sees (or knows about) his friends carrying on with their lives and moving on without him. He feels unloved and unimportant. He is now a nobody.
   - He feels socially isolated.

8. *What does it mean to feel socially isolated?*
   - It is more than being lonely. Tim meets no one at all apart from his family. When people go to school or work they interact with

many people, which gives interest to the day and allows many small rewarding conversations to take place.

- It is possible to feel lonely and socially isolated even when there are many people around you, as you can mentally and emotionally cut yourself off from others making it impossible for them to 'reach' you. Then you don't experience others' feelings of care for you or your feelings for them.

- When people feel socially isolated they lose their sense of worth and importance in the world and can very easily become depressed.

9. (a) *Many chronically sick people suffer from depression. What is this?*

Depression is a feeling of deep unhappiness that doesn't leave you. You may feel so low that you do not want to get out of bed at all, lose all interest in yourself and do not eat properly or wash. The intensity of your unhappiness is so great that you cannot 'snap out of it', but many people may tell you to, thinking that you only need a strong talking-to.

Other symptoms of depression include tiredness, pessimism, feelings of hopelessness and sometimes anxiety, loss of appetite and weight and insomnia. It is common to have suicidal feelings and there is a high risk of suicide in the depressed – that is why it is essential to seek medical help.

(b) *Other people suffer from depression too. Can you give some examples?*

Sometimes something definite causes depression, such as a prolonged illness or a tragic life event (being a victim of a crime or suffering bereavement), and sometimes it has grown with you through an unhappy childhood. Sometimes the cause is not known. Depression is common with people suffering from the following:

- child abuse
- chronic illnesses
- eating disorders
- feelings of inadequacy and not being able to cope following the birth of a baby (post-natal depression)
- obsessive–compulsive disorders

- phobias and panic attacks
- post-traumatic stress
- redundancy and unemployment.

10. What can be done to help a depressed person?

- He or she could be offered counselling.

- He or she could be given medication called an anti-depressant. There are many different types working in slightly different ways so that usually one can be found to suit.

- It is helpful to get out and meet people and go out with friends. (However, this is not possible with people who are housebound through old age, illness or disability. Also, people who cannot get out and about tend to have less in common with those who do and so conversation can be difficult. This is why people tend to lose their friends when they stop work, or are unable to attend school.)

STORY 27: *Hands Off!*

Harriet worked two evenings a week at a late night chemist's. She needed the money as her parents could not afford to give her pocket money and, as she had hopes of becoming a pharmacist herself, she wanted some relevant experience.

The first few times Mr Eagles, her boss, brushed past her, Harriet thought nothing of it – she just assumed he was too busy to wait for her to pass out of the back of the shop before he went in. But now he kept putting his arm around her, pulling her to him until his fingers reached under her breast and Harriet felt unable to move away.

She wished she could leave and find a job somewhere else, but could she rely on Mr Eagles to give her a good reference? How would she explain her reasons for leaving? She had to do something as her boss was now finding more reasons for her to be at the back of the shop with him and his hands were moving to more intimate places...

'You must have been encouraging him,' Tania told her.

'I have not!' Harriet denied hotly.

'Well, why didn't you stop him? I wouldn't let anyone feel me up!'

'I don't know – I wasn't sure at first, and then it was too late.'

Some boys in the class had overheard their conversation. 'Harriet's a slag,' they said to everyone who was close enough to hear. 'Bet she's already pregnant, so she's making up stories to put the blame on someone else.'

'With a body like hers, she can't be too picky. I expect she thought she'd better take what was on offer – it would be her only chance!'

'Hey, Harriet! What was it like? You should try it with someone younger – granddads have no stamina!'

'I bet the first time was her last time. She tried it and didn't like it. With boobs like hers, she's just got to be a lesbian!'

'Prefer girls, do you Harriet? Watch out Tania, she'll have her hands wandering all over you next, now she knows how to do it!'

Harriet felt hurt and was furious that people could say such things to her. Friends should support her, not make things even harder. However, she knew they wanted her to react to them, so she didn't. 'You may not know it, but you've all just done me a great favour. I now know I'm the only person I can truly rely on. Me. And I know what to do.'

The next time Harriet was at work, she waited for a quiet moment when there weren't any customers. 'Mr Eagles, I enjoy working here, but I don't feel comfortable with you touching me – in any way at all. If it happens again, I'll phone your wife and the regional manager. I have kept a diary of what has happened while I've been working here and I have told my parents. And if you hurt me in any way, I'll go to the police. Do you believe me?'

Mr Eagles spluttered as though he were going to deny having touched her in a way that was inappropriate, but catching her steely eyes and seeing the determined lift of her chin, he thought better of it. Slowly, he nodded. He did understand.

Discussion Sheet 27: Hands Off!

1. The main theme of this story is sexual harassment. What is it?

2. (a) Explain why Harriet hadn't tried to stop Mr Eagles' advances when they first started.

   (b) What effect did this have on Mr Eagles?

3. Have you been sexually harassed (boys and girls)? Have you sexually harassed someone else? If so, what happened?

4. Do you agree with how Harriet handled the situation with Mr Eagles? Might she have been in danger from him, or do you think confronting him about his behaviour lessened the possibility of her coming to harm?

5. (a) Sometimes, teachers are sexually harassed by their pupils. For example, a pupil might spread unfounded rumours that a female teacher is pregnant or ask very personal questions out of the context of the lesson.

Are women teachers less human, an 'easy' target or less able than their male colleagues?

(b) Why do they get harassed?

(c) Why do pupils harass teachers (male and female)?

6. Are women 'equal' to men? If they are, why do they not have the same status in most areas of life?

7. (a) Sexual harassment is a form of bullying. An extreme form of it is rape, when the harasser is male. It has been reported that some teenage boys rape teenage girls. Can you account for their attitudes towards women?

(b) How have they become like this at such a young age?

8. (a) Have you been brought up to believe that women are second-class citizens?

(b) What myths support this idea?

9. Do you support sexist attitudes, let them by without comment or confront them? (Boys and girls.) Or do you consider that feminist attitudes to sexism are exaggerated and have no relevance to you?

10. What can *you* do to stamp out sexism and sexual harassment in men and women?

Leader Sheet 27: Hands Off!

1. **The main theme of this story is sexual harassment. What is it?**

   - Sexual harassment is any unwanted and uninvited sexual attention that undermines your confidence in yourself and your work. In the workplace it can prevent you doing your job properly, creates a stressful environment and threatens your job security or chances of a promotion.

   - Sexual harassment is any behaviour that makes you feel uncomfortable, embarrassed, compromised or ill at ease.

   - It can involve touching, pinching, standing too close, talking straight into your face, rubbing up against you, physical assault or rape, verbal assaults – sexual innuendo, jokes, comments on appearance, sexual propositions and emotional blackmail. It also includes offensive use of pin-ups, pornographic pictures and patronising language.

2. **(a) Explain why Harriet hadn't tried to stop Mr Eagles' advances when they first started.**

   Harriet assumed he was too busy to wait for her to pass out of the back of the shop before he went in. She thought it was completely innocent.

   (b) What effect did this have on Mr Eagles?

   It gave him encouragement to become bolder because she hadn't protested. He decided to take advantage of her silence.

3. **Have you been sexually harassed (boys and girls)? Have you sexually harassed someone else? If so, what happened?**

   (Personal responses required.)

4. **Do you agree with how Harriet handled the situation with Mr Eagles? Might she have been in danger from him, or do you think confronting him about his behaviour lessened the possibility of her coming to harm?**

   There was no evidence to suggest she would be in danger from him – he hadn't threatened her or told her not to tell anyone. However, you can never be certain. But everyone knew that she was working with him at that time so if she disappeared, he would be the first person her parents and police would question. And since she claimed she had already told her parents what had happened and had kept a diary there would be hard evidence. If he believed this, it would probably keep her safe.

Because Harriet reacted so swiftly and strongly as soon as she realised what was going on, she probably gave him a shock that stopped him in his tracks. She also told him what she would do if he didn't leave her alone. Because she gave him a get-out ('If you do this again I'll...') he was not completely cornered. He was safe from being exposed as long as he behaved himself with her.

5. **(a) Sometimes, teachers are sexually harassed by their pupils. For example, a pupil might spread unfounded rumours that a female teacher is pregnant or ask very personal questions out of the context of the lesson. Are women teachers less human, an 'easy' target or less able than their male colleagues?**

- Women teachers are not less human but they may be seen as an easy target as they are not traditionally associated with heavy discipline. They may also be smaller than the pupils they teach whereas many men would be taller and stockier, creating a stronger presence in the classroom.

- Some pupils, because they have been brought up in a sexist environment, may think that women teachers are less intelligent, and therefore less worthy of their good behaviour.

- Some pupils might not take women teachers seriously when they say things like, 'If you do that one more time I'll...' because they have experienced inconsistent discipline from their mother at home.

- In primary schools women teachers predominate, particularly in infant schools. The higher up in the school system you go, there is a trend for a greater proportion of male teachers. This may give pupils the message that women teachers are not that capable of handling older children.

- Women teachers are definitely not less able than men teachers – although pupils from some backgrounds may not accept this. For example, boys from some Muslim backgrounds may not accept authority from a woman or give her the same respect as they would a man.

(b) Why do they get harassed?

- Because the children are bored and see women teachers as an easy target, for the reasons suggested above.

- Because boys are fascinated by the opposite sex's sexuality. They may say things like 'Smile if you had it off last night,' or if a teacher wears clothing that accentuates her abdomen, the pupils (girls and boys) might ask her if she was pregnant and pass rumours around the school to that effect.

(c) Why do pupils harass teachers (male and female)?

- Because they detect something about the teacher that stands out as being different from the expected norms (stereotypes). For example, an effeminate man would be an immediate target for harassment. A butch woman equally so.

- To relieve boredom.

- Because young people naturally fight against authority, constantly wanting to check and challenge boundaries. If they perceive any form of vulnerability or weakness in a teacher they will make use of it.

6. Are women 'equal' to men? If they are, why do they not have the same status in most areas of life?

Women are equal to men but social attitudes towards women's place in society need to change. For example:

- If an employer is sexist they might choose to promote a man over a woman to a high level position because they want to avoid a highly responsible employee having time off work to have children.

- Women may be thought of as less reliable than men, having mood swings (pre-menstrual tension) and needing time off when they have their periods.

- Women are generally paid less than men doing the same job and have to be that much better in order to be given the job over a man in the first place.

- In many faiths, women are regarded as inferior to men.
- In some cultures, women are not allowed to own land.

This unfair treatment of women is to do with sexism: treating people differently depending on whether they are male or female in the belief that women are inferior to men. Sexism suits the need, which many men feel, to dominate in society. Many men intimidate women and fight against their struggle for equality in order to retain their domination. However, not all men or organisations are sexist.

7. (a) *Sexual harassment is a form of bullying. An extreme form of it is rape, when the harasser is male. It has been reported that some teenage boys rape teenage girls. Can you account for their attitudes towards women?*

- Some boys do not believe that a girl or woman really means it when she says 'no' (for example to sex). This provides them with an excuse to have intercourse anyway. Often rape in these circumstances is 'date rape', where the girl has gone out with a boy and he forces her to have sex. It is then difficult to prove that rape has occurred.
- Some boys may feel the need to dominate or subjugate a girl and get a thrill out of it, making them feel powerful and in control.
- Some boys abuse their superior strength by raping girls for their own pleasure, without having to work hard at developing a mutually loving relationship.

(b) *How have they become like this at such a young age?*

- If boys are brought up in a sexist society and they hear sexist comments in the home and witness sexist behaviour, they too are likely to view girls as play things, to be used or abused.
- Perhaps the rapists have been sexually abused themselves and so they repeat the experience on someone more vulnerable than themselves.

8. (a) *Have you been brought up to believe that women are second-class citizens?*

(Personal response required.)

(b) What myths support this idea?

- Expressions such as, 'A woman's place is in the home'; 'To keep a woman under control, keep her barefoot and pregnant'.
- Assumptions such as women being natural mothers and child-carers; the best person to do domestic chores and chores disliked by men (such as cleaning toilets).
- Expecting women to be 'the weaker sex'.

9. Do you support sexist attitudes, let them by without comment or confront them? (Boys and girls.) Or do you consider that feminist attitudes to sexism are exaggerated and have no relevance to you?

(Personal responses required.)

10. What can you do to stamp out sexism and sexual harassment directed towards men and women?

To stamp out sexism towards men:

- Point out the unfairness of a situation when it happens. For example, some young boys are not allowed to play with dolls and dress up in girls' clothes for fear that they may adopt feminine traits. This is denying them the opportunity to explore their world in an open way.
- When someone makes a sexist joke in your hearing (such as poking fun at men's inability to cook or clean as well as their female counterparts), defend youe sex. 'Your partner may not be able to cook or clean as well as you, but it doesn't mean that all men share these characteristics and I feel offended that you think they do'
- If someone asks you to do something within your stereotype, challenge the person. For example, if you are the only man present and you are asked to help a woman whose car's broken down, you could say, 'Why presume I know more about car maintenance than you?'

To stamp out sexism towards women:

- Point out the unfairness of a situation or of what someone has said every time it happens. For example, if you are expected to be out at work all day and then come home and do the cleaning, ironing and cooking when your partner works the same number of hours, you should insist on sharing the tasks equally. If you are still at school and are studying for exams and your older brother is at home, you should protest about having to do domestic chores while your brother does nothing merely because he is male.

- When someone makes a sexist joke in your hearing you could point out that you find it offensive or make it obvious from your body language that you do not appreciate the humour.

- If someone asks you to do something within your stereotype, check their reasons first. For example, if you are asked to take notes in a discussion group where you're the only girl and you believe the others are assigning secretarial duties to you because they see it as a fitting job for you, challenge them. Ask, 'Did you ask me to do this because I'm female or because you think I'm good at taking notes?'

To stamp out sexual harassment towards men:

- If you are a man at work, who is being sexually harassed by a woman, make your position clear to her and, if she doesn't stop, take it to personnel and insist they take your complaint seriously. (This is stressed as, traditionally, male sterotyping is such that men are expected to cope with women and 'keep them in their place'. Another male stereotype is the expectation that men are predatory and will accept advances from any willing female. This is patently incorrect and men can make their position clear to all witnesses.)

To stamp out sexual harassment towards women:

- You should rebuff any unwelcome overtures a man makes towards you and complain to his face, or to your head of section (or personnel), if he makes sexist jokes or innuendoes in your hearing while at work.

To stamp out sexual harassment towards either sex:

- If going to personnel doesn't work or you feel unable to approach staff in authority, try to get witnesses to events and keep a diary of what the person does and says. This can provide evidence if you later need it. Putting up with sexual harassment does not make it stop.

- If you are still at school, you should approach your form teacher or Head of Year.

STORY 28: He Was My Boyfriend!

'I'll miss you while I'm away', Rhian told Declan, her boyfriend of one year. She knew she was going to miss him desperately. Three weeks was going to seem like forever. Rhian also felt sorry for her best friend, Lorna, who had no brothers or sisters and relied on her for company and for going out. Lately, Lorna had been joining her and Declan if they went bowling or ice-skating.

'I'll miss you too,' Declan replied, kissing her nose.

'I hope Lorna doesn't get too lonely while I'm gone,' Rhian mused.

'Don't worry. I'll be around if she's desperate.'

Rhian smiled. 'Thanks. You're so understanding.'

'Declan? It's Lorna. I wondered if you fancied going to see that new film. I knew you would probably be at a loose end with Rhian being away and thought we could keep each other company.'

Declan wondered if going to the cinema was what Rhian had in mind when she wanted him to look after her friend. Well, it would do no harm. And, afterall, why shouldn't he go? – Rhian was enjoying herself.

'Yeah. That's a good idea. Where do we meet and when?'

Three weeks later, Rhian was home. The first thing she did after unpacking was to ring Declan. But he wasn't there. And his mum had sounded strange.

Rhian then phoned Lorna, to see if she was free that evening. But she wasn't there either. And her mother sounded strained when she asked her about her holiday.

Thinking that Declan would be over as soon as his mum told him she was back, Rhian decided to shower and wash her hair so that she looked her best. She had quite a good tan too, despite wearing sun-block.

Later that evening, the doorbell rang. But it wasn't only Declan who was there – Lorna was with him.

'Hi!' Rhian said brightly. 'What a coincidence for both of you to turn up at the same time! Come in.' Her face fell as she saw Declan and Lorna exchange glances. They looked very uncomfortable about something.

'There's something we have to tell you,' Lorna said.

We? Rhian asked herself. We? Lorna and Declan?

'What do you want to say?' Rhian asked huskily. She had a good idea but wanted to hear it from them. There was no reason why she should make it easy for them.

'I'm sorry, Rhian,' Lorna began, ' but while you were away, Declan and I saw a lot of each other.'

'And?'

'And we've fallen for each other,' Lorna whispered. Declan took hold of her hand.

Rhian could barely stand the pain but had to know more. 'How did it happen?'

Lorna shrugged. 'It just did. We went out together and realised we were having great fun and that we clicked. It sort of snowballed from there.'

'I thought you were my friend. I trusted you, Lorna. Declan was *my* boyfriend and you took him away.'

'She didn't take me away. I wanted to go. It would have happened sooner or later anyway,' Declan told her.

Rhian felt betrayed by both of them. She'd lost her best friend and boyfriend in one go. She felt shamed and rejected. She hadn't known there was anything wrong between her and Declan – and hadn't even had a chance to put things right.

Discussion Sheet 28: He Was My Boyfriend!

1. Do you agree that 'All is fair in love…'? That if you like someone you can do anything to get him or her, even when the person is with someone else?

2. (a) Is taking someone else's partner away from someone OK as long as he or she is not married?

   (b) Or does marriage make no difference to your answer?

3. How do you think this experience will affect Rhian in future relationships?

4. (a) How do you think Rhian felt, knowing her partner had left her for someone else?

   (b) Has this happened to you?

5. How do you think Rhian felt towards Lorna now?

6. Rhian had had no warning that Declan wasn't happy in the relationship. If he had wanted to split up with her anyway what would have been a better way to go about it?

7. Was Declan telling the truth about their break-up happening sooner or later and that he'd wanted to leave?

8. Have you taken a partner away from a friend or made someone else's best friend into your best friend? What happened? How did the other person react?

9. Are teenage romances as important as adult ones?

10. Whose betrayal was worse? Lorna's or Declan's? Why?

Leader Sheet 28: He Was My Boyfriend!

1. ***Do you agree that 'All is fair in love...'? That if you like someone you can do anything to get him or her, even when the person is with someone else?***

   Yes: The person isn't likely to stay with the same partner forever when in his or her teens. You should make your feelings clear to the person you've fallen for and hope that he or she will feel the same – with a little help.

   No: It's just an excuse people use when they betray someone they were close to and who trusted them. It's supposed to make them feel better about what they've done – even justify it. It's saying that what you did is OK because you're madly in love and it is meant to be – but it's not OK.

   It would be very wrong to try to take someone away from his or her partner deliberately. You can't do just anything and think it's OK.

2. ***(a) Is taking someone else's partner away from someone OK as long as he or she is not married?***

   (Personal response required.)

   Please note, this question refers to one person *deliberately* trying to split up a couple. It is not intended to cast judgement where marriages or relationships have failed for any other reason, such as immense mutual attraction between the people concerned.

   (b) Or does marriage make no difference to your answer?

   Marriage should make a difference to your response. Two people have committed themselves to loving each other above all others for life and that should be respected. If someone is married, you should leave well alone. A man or woman who can easily contemplate being unfaithful to his or her partner once you've shown how you feel is not likely to worry about being faithful to you or your needs. Plus it is unkind to the person's partner. It is worse if children are involved as the divorce or separation that can follow such unfaithfulness can cause immense distress.

3. ***How do you think this experience will affect Rhian in future relationships?***

She might:

- become over-possessive of future boyfriends
- find it hard to trust either boyfriends or girlfriends again
- be unable to commit herself emotionally for fear of getting hurt
- have nothing more to do with Lorna
- develop new friendships with both sexes and use her wariness to monitor closely how her relationship is faring.

4. ***(a) How do you think Rhian felt, knowing her partner had left her for someone else?***

- A target for jokes.
- Betrayed.
- Disbelieving.
- Hurt.
- Rejected.
- Sad.
- Shamed.
- Unloved.

(b) Has this happened to you?

(Personal response required.)

5. ***How do you think Rhian felt towards Lorna now?***

- Angry.
- Bitter.
- Hating.
- Vengeful (wanting to get her own back).

6. ***Rhian had had no warning that Declan wasn't happy in the relationship. If he had wanted to split up with her anyway what would have been a better way to go about it?***

- He could first have tried to put things right by explaining what was lacking in their relationship and by talking about what they could do to improve things. This would also have given Rhian an opportunity to say some things of her own that she would like changed and they would both reach a better understanding of the other.

- If this didn't work, or he simply had lost his feelings for Rhian or no longer enjoyed her company, Declan could have told her that the relationship was no longer working for him and could they just be friends? This lets her down more gently and gives her the opportunity to maintain contact with him and carry on enjoying his company – perhaps in a group rather than as a couple. This is important as neither might want to lose the friendship of the other.

- Breaking up in stages (showing irritation or dissatisfaction or a gradual cool-off) so that Rhian knows something is wrong and is let down gently.

7. Was Declan telling the truth about their break-up happening sooner or later and that he'd wanted to leave?

Teenage relationships don't often survive well into adulthood so they probably would have split up sometime – this part was true. However, this does not mean that his and Rhian's relationship was on the verge of breaking up. He hadn't wanted to leave the relationship when she went away. He seemed reluctant at first to go out with Lorna and he felt guilty because he was going to the cinema with her and not perhaps somewhere less intimate such as going out for a drink. It was obvious that Lorna had made a play for him as she was the lonely one.

8. Have you taken a partner away from a friend or made someone else's best friend into your best friend? What happened? How did the other person react?

(Personal responses required.)

9. Are teenage romances as important as adult ones?

Yes:

- They provide much learning experience about people and relationships. Without the clumsy handling of early relationships and the angst of betrayal and losing someone you love, you are less prepared for adult romances.

- By the time you have had a few relationships, you are more clued-up about what qualities you want in a partner. And you realise that the ideal partner does not exist. Life is full of compromise. (But that doesn't mean you should compromise your values and accept any behaviour – such as abusive behaviour.)

No:

- They are not as vital as adult ones. The consequences are rarely as big since teenage relationships don't involve children, having responsibility for paying bills and rent or paying a mortgage, or making a lifelong commitment and then having to break it.
- They tend to be small trial-and-error relationships where you learn more about people as you are growing up.

10. Whose betrayal was worse? Lorna's or Declan's? Why?

Lorna's was worse:

- She was Rhian's best friend and best friend relationships should survive the comings and goings of the partners in their lives.
- Because best friends are special, you are closest to them and trust them the most with all your secrets and problems.
- Lorna had been invited along with the two of them out of Rhian's kindness. It was no way to repay her thoughtfulness.
- You might have had years and years of history between you and your best friend and betrayal destroys the memory of all the things you'd shared together.
- Losing a best friend can be like losing a partner in adult life.

Declan's was worse:

- He had probably told Rhian that he loved her – they had been going out for a year. So the betrayal makes Rhian feel as though she'd been lied to and that he hadn't been honest with her all along. It will destroy her trust in other boys.
- It was also like a slap in the face for Rhian to have him prefer her best friend, particularly when Lorna had tagged along so often at Rhian's suggestion.

STORY 29: SIDA

Hannah had invited her friend, Donna, to her house for the first time one Saturday afternoon. They went straight up to Hannah's room.

'Don't you have a CD player?' Donna asked.

'No, but I've got a radio/cassette recorder. I'll put some music on.'

'That's not very loud. Don't they let you play loud music?'

'Yes, but at the moment Mum's not well, so I don't want to disturb her.'

'What's wrong with her?'

'Some kind of flu,' Hannah replied, looking out of her window. She wished she had a friend she could confide in; trust. 'Would you like to see my scrapbook?'

'What sort of scrapbook?'

'A family one. Look.' Hannah brought down a bulging hard-backed book from her shelf. It was full of photographs with a full paragraph of writing under each, describing the day and what they did. 'This was last Christmas, when we had our Grandma and Grandpa to stay. And this was my last birthday.'

Donna felt embarrassed. It seemed a bit heavy, mooning over family photographs. She'd expected an album of pop stars. Hannah was weird. 'What are those tapes up there?' she asked, changing the subject.

'Those are the recordings made at Christmas times and birthdays and so on.' Hannah didn't want to share those with anyone. They were for herself only.

'Oh,' Donna replied. Surely Hannah wasn't going to expect her to listen to any of them? 'What do you do in your spare time?'

'I help look after Mum and do my scrapbook and make tapes. And listen to music.'

'You did say she had flu didn't you? That doesn't last that long, surely?'

'No,' Hannah agreed quietly. 'She does get ill a lot though. She's got a weak immune system.'

'Has she got cancer?' Donna asked sympathetically.

Hannah took a deep breath. She needed to talk to someone her own age about it. 'No. AIDS.'

'What?'

'AIDS.'

Donna recoiled in horror. It was the sort of disease other people had, but not someone you knew about. She was terrified. Suppose she caught it?

'She got it from a blood transfusion, before they'd started to screen against AIDS,' Hannah told her, not wanting Donna to think her mum had been promiscuous.

An embarrassed silence fell between them. Hannah regretted telling and Donna wondered how quickly she could make her excuses and go home.

'Would you like a drink? I've made some cookies,' Hannah offered.

'Thanks, but I'm not thirsty or hungry. But I do need the toilet. Where is it?'

Hannah told her, recognising her friend's emotional withdrawal. Perhaps Donna thought she had AIDS too?

Donna was very careful not to touch the toilet seat and flushed the chain by holding onto some tissue before letting it fall into the bowl. When she washed her hands, she shook them dry, not wanting to touch any towels.

When Donna got back, Hannah said, 'I've upset you, haven't I? You're scared of catching it.'

There didn't seem any point in lying. 'Yes, I am,' she admitted. 'Have you got it?'

'No. And you won't either. Dad has but that's because they had sex without knowing Mum had it. But they're careful now so that they don't swap different strains of HIV – it can change in your body. We'll probably be grown up before Dad gets ill – if not we can be fostered. We're a bit old for adoption now and we don't want it.'

Donna looked closely at Hannah and wondered if *she'd* have coped so well knowing she would lose both parents. She doubted it.

Discussion Sheet 29: SIDA

1. What does AIDS stand for? What is it?

2. What does it mean, to be HIV positive?

3. List ways in which you can become infected with HIV.

4. List ways in which you can interact or live with a person but stand no risk of catching HIV.

5. How would you (or do you) feel about someone you know who is HIV positive? If you knew the person before he or she caught HIV, would you change towards him or her in any way? If so, in what ways and why? Are the reasons rational? (This may depend on the type of relationship you have.)

6. (a) Do you know what health problems an HIV-positive person faces?

   (b) Has someone close to you died from an AIDS-related illness? If so, how did you feel about it?

7. If now, or in the future, there is a remote possibility that you may have intercourse with someone, would you carry condoms 'just in case'? If not, why not?

8. Where can you obtain free condoms (and in some cases free Femidoms)?

9. (a) Has the issue of HIV scared you? Are you afraid, because of the risk of HIV, of forming sexual relationships?

   (b) If so, how can you reduce this anxiety?

   (c) Do you think a potential partner should tell you of known HIV positiveness?

   (d) If so, at what stage would you expect or hope this to happen?

10. Anonymity of HIV-positive people is preserved in work-places and schools. Do you agree with this or do you feel you have a right to know who is HIV positive in your class or workplace? Think of both sides of the argument.

Leader Sheet 29: SIDA

1. What does AIDS stand for? What is it?

AIDS stands for Acquired Immune Deficiency Syndrome and is the name for different diseases that can cause serious illness or death as a result of infection by the Human Immunodeficiency Virus (HIV) which damages the body's immune system.

2. What does it mean, to be HIV positive?

It means the person has HIV antibodies in his or her bloodstream. It can take at least three months for HIV antibodies to produce a positive result after infection – and during this time the person is infectious. It can take 10 to 15 years for HIV to destroy the body's immune system – it is not known if everyone with HIV will die. Babies can carry their mother's HIV antibodies for 18 months after birth and then be tested negative – in these cases the babies are HIV free.

3. List ways in which you can become infected with HIV.

HIV can be transmitted:

- through body fluid spills. Splashes in the eye or mouth can transmit the virus. (HIV is present in blood, semen and vaginal secretions; and is present in minute quantities in tears and saliva, but these are insufficient to cause infection. It is not present in urine, vomit, stools or nasal mucus unless blood is also present.)

- through unprotected penetrative sex, with the penis entering the vagina, rectum or mouth (this is less risky). If the person has mouth ulcers, sores or a sore throat, the virus is given ready access to the person's bloodstream.

- more easily if either partner has a sexually transmitted disease – these leave people more vulnerable to the risk of infection by weakening the immune system and the sores and ulcers that may occur offer a ready route of entry to the virus.

- more easily to the man during intercourse with a menstruating woman, although transmission can occur at other times if vaginal secretions enter the hole at the end of the penis. Transmission from man to woman is twice as likely as from woman to man.

- through the sharing of needles and syringes and through any infected blood products reaching the bloodstream.
- from mother to foetus or to baby by breast-feeding – although only about one in five or six babies born to HIV-positive mothers in the UK and Europe will be affected. Bottle-feeding can reduce risks.
- through the use of unsterilised ear piercing, tattooing and acupuncture equipment that has previously been used on a person with the HIV virus.
- theoretically through sharing toothbrushes and razors, as could having oral sex immediately after brushing teeth as the gums may bleed and provide a ready route for the virus.
- from dried blood on a towel, as HIV may survive on it for five or six days. But the quantities of virus that enter someone's bloodstream may be insufficient to cause infection.

HIV cannot survive in very hot water, bleach or detergent. (But to re-use syringes if no new ones are available, they must be rinsed twice with cold water, then twice with bleach solution and then twice with cold water again. Hot water clots the blood.)

4. *List ways in which you can interact or live with a person but stand no risk of catching HIV.*

HIV cannot be transmitted through:

- animals or pets
- coughing
- eating food prepared by an HIV-positive person
- mosquitoes and other insects
- sharing a drinking fountain
- sharing a toilet seat
- showers
- sneezing
- sweat
- swimming pools (the water treatment kills the virus – and even if it didn't, it would be so diluted as to be present in insufficient quantity to infect the person)

- tears.

It is only present in body fluids – blood, semen, breast milk, menstrual fluid, vaginal secretions. (It is present in vomit and stools only when there is blood in them from illness.)

5. *How would you (or do you) feel about someone you know who is HIV positive? If you knew the person before he or she caught HIV, would you change towards him or her in any way? If so, in what ways and why? Are the reasons rational? (This may depend on the type of relationship you have.)*

(Personal responses required.)

6. *(a) Do you know what health problems an HIV-positive person faces?*

At first, after being infected with HIV, the person may experience mild flu-like symptoms. Then the virus may be relatively inactive for several years and the person feels quite well. But as the virus multiplies it weakens the immune system and the person becomes vulnerable to infections and conditions that do not usually trouble those with a healthy immune system.

The person is not considered to have AIDS until he or she develops at least one serious infection from a special list made up by the Centers for Disease Control in the USA. Even if the person is extremely unwell with a particular illness, unless it is on the list he or she is still not classed as having AIDS. Instead, it would be called an HIV-related illness.

HIV-related illnesses include:

- herpes simplex infections (cold sores)
- oral thrush
- salmonellosis
- shingles
- skin inflammation, particularly affecting the face
- tuberculosis.

The commonest symptoms of AIDS-related conditions are a worsening of the above symptoms of thrush and herpes simplex and:

- extreme fatigue lasting up to several weeks with no apparent cause
- fever and night sweats

- prolonged diarrhoea
- prolonged shortness of breath and a dry cough
- skin disease – pink or purple blotches on the skin or eyelids. They are usually hard and look like a bruise or blood blister
- swollen glands, especially in the neck and armpits
- unexpected weight loss.

AIDS-related illnesses include:

- auto-immune diseases (where a reaction of the person's immune system acts against his or her own organs and body tissues)
- cancers
- pneumonia and other severe infections
- toxoplasmosis (an infection that can be caught from cats).

(b) Has someone close to you died from an AIDS-related illness? If so, how did you feel about it?

(Personal responses required.)

7. *If now, or in the future, there is a remote possibility that you may have intercourse with someone, would you carry condoms 'just in case'? If not, why not?*

(Personal responses required.)

8. *Where can you obtain free condoms (and in some cases free Femidoms)?*

Family planning clinics. You do not even have to be seen by a doctor.

9. *(a) Has the issue of HIV scared you? Are you afraid, because of the risk of HIV, of forming sexual relationships?*

(Personal responses required.)

(b) If so, how can you reduce this anxiety?

- By not being promiscuous.
- By ensuring that the boy or man *always* wears a condom. (This ensures that semen does not enter your body.)
- Many people are unaware that they have HIV antibodies so one can never assume that a partner is clear of HIV infection. The only way to make sure is for both potential partners to be tested – and

this is done with complete confidentiality at STD (sexually transmitted diseases) clinics.

(c) Do you think a potential partner should tell you of known HIV positiveness?

Yes, because he or she would be risking your life.

(d) If so, at what stage would you expect or hope this to happen?

Before sexual intercourse takes place. And not immediately before – as soon as the relationship has become intimate so that you have time to think about the consequences and absorb the information. You could be given an opportunity to receive reassurance or counselling from a professional to make informed decisions.

10. Anonymity of HIV-positive people is preserved in workplaces and schools. Do you agree with this or do you feel you have a right to know who is HIV positive in your class or workplace? Think of both sides of the argument.

For preserving anonymity:

- People are still ignorant about how you can catch HIV so they would avoid you if they knew you had it.
- People might tell everyone else and label you as being HIV positive rather than recognising you as a person.
- Friends might not invite you to their homes because their families would be afraid of catching it.
- The issue is not preserving anonymity but educating people about how to look after themselves. If they are told that one person has it but not another because that person doesn't know himself, it would give them a false sense of security and they would not behave safely.

Against preserving anonymity:

- You'd want to know whether you have to be careful if your friend has got HIV and they cut themselves. (Note: Not everyone knows they have HIV or hepatitis, for example, so you should be careful of anyone's body fluids in any case.)
- You have a right to know from whom you are at risk.
- If you knew the numbers of HIV-infected people, you might take the risks of unprotected sex more seriously.

STORY 30: 2052 AD

I'm Jane and this is my story about smoking.

I was told with the rest of my class at school not to smoke, but I thought I knew better. Even though the consequences of my smoking were laid out in front of me, I thought they did not apply to me. I thought I could rise above them.

I was convinced that by the time I wanted a family I would be able to give up. Easily. But I couldn't and that's why I'm guarded 24 hours a day and my visitors are searched.

You see, it's the right of the unborn child to develop free from the harmful effects of tobacco smoke. I filled in a form when I first wanted a licence to buy cigarettes and signed an agreement to accept government regulations.

Treatment for illnesses or diseases related to tobacco smoke are no longer funded by the health service. And if pregnant mothers fail a test to check for tobacco smoke then they are installed in a special wing of hospitals at their own expense to ensure that their unborn child is protected.

I've had to take out a loan for my confinement. It will take me a long time to pay it back. Also, it's very boring spending so many months in the same building.

If, knowing you cannot give up smoking, you hide a pregnancy from the authorities, you forfeit the right even to know your baby after he or she has been born. I did not want to risk this but, also, I want what's best for my child. I don't want to give her a legacy of possible illnessess or – indeed her own children, if it's a girl. And I'm used to not smoking now. I know I shall never start again.

Robbie, my partner, however, is a heavy smoker and so far has been unable to drop the habit. With only four weeks to go until my baby's birth, he's cutting it fine. I'm feeling very frustrated and angry with him. I've had to stop so why can't he?

You see, children aren't allowed to be brought up in a smoky atmosphere after they've been born. So if Robbie continues to smoke, I lose my child. I cannot afford to set up home on my own. And I really don't want my baby fostered.

As I'm getting to the end of my pregnancy, I find that I'm getting more and more attached to my bump. And less attached to Robbie.

I now know that I want my baby more than I want him.

Discussion Sheet 30: 2052 AD

1. (a) Should unborn babies and children have the right to grow in a smoke-free atmosphere?

   (b) If yes, should the government enforce this as suggested in the story?

   (c) Why does Jane say she now wants her baby more than Robbie?

2. (a) What are the negative effects of smoking on the body?

   (b) What chemicals are in cigarettes?

3. Would you give up smoking if you were knowingly going to try for a baby? (This applies to boys too.)

4. Should children sue parents or guardians who are responsible for their developing smoking-related illnesses through passive smoking?

5. If your home is smoky, are there negotiations you can make with the smokers to keep some areas free from smoke, for your health and the health of your pets?

6. Will there come a time when there is an official policy for smoking-related illnesses *not* to be treated on the NHS (UK National Health Service)?

7. Is it fair that non-smoking tax-payers foot the bill for self-induced illnesses such as from tobacco smoking? Should the tobacco companies themselves have to pay? Or should the government use only the amount they gain from taxes on tobacco to treat patients?

8. (a) Why do people smoke?

   (b) Why do people choose not to smoke?

   (c) What are the effects of giving up smoking on the body?

9. Should smoking be banned in public and workplaces to avoid 'passive' smoking?

10. Should tobacco companies sponsor sports events, thus giving smoking a 'healthy' image?

Leader Sheet 30: 2052 AD

1. **(a) *Should unborn babies and children have the right to grow in a smoke-free atmosphere?***

Yes – but there is no one to uphold this except the mother in the case of the unborn child and the parents and guardians for born children.

(b) *If yes, should the government enforce this as suggested in the story?*

(Personal response required.)

(c) *Why does Jane say she now wants her baby more than Robbie?*

Robbie doesn't look as though he's going to manage to give up smoking. Jane has to choose between keeping her baby and staying with Robbie – she can't have both as Robbie smokes.

2. **(a) *What are the negative effects of smoking on the body?***

- Narrowing of blood vessels, increased heart rate and blood pressure and reduction in urine output.
- First-time users often feel dizzy and nauseated and may even vomit.
- A smoker's cough or shortness of breath are early signs of lung damage or heart disease.
- Women are at greater risk of getting cancer of the cervix and they are more likely to reach the menopause two to three years early.
- Cigarette smoking reduces the blood levels of a variety of drugs and reduces their effects.
- Diabetics may need larger doses of insulin, and the health risks involved in taking oral contraceptives are increased by smoking.

Diseases caused by smoking include:

- Cancer of the lungs and bronchus (main airway tube), mouth, nose, throat, larynx (voice box), oesophagus (tube that takes your food to your stomach), pancreas, bladder, cervix, kidneys and blood (leukaemia).

- Heart disease, atherosclerosis (build-up of fat in arteries that reduces the elasticity in the artery walls) which can lead to strokes (these risks are greatly increased if the person is also taking oral contraceptives), gangrene (legs, for example, may need to be amputated due to a reduced blood supply) and thinning of arteries (aneurisms).
- Osteoporosis, leading to brittle bones.
- Recurrent infections of the lungs and airways, chronic bronchitis and emphysema (loss of elasticity and efficiency in the lungs leading to lack of oxygen in the person's body which can create other medical problems – and he or she has difficulty breathing).
- Peptic ulcers (due to excess production of stomach acid) in the stomach and duodenum.
- Reduced fertility.

(b) What chemicals are in cigarettes?

Each cigarette contains over 4000 chemicals including:

- ammonia – which is found in household cleaners
- butane – used to fuel lighters and tar
- carbon monoxide – the lethal gas that comes out of car exhausts
- cyanide and arsenic – which are poisons
- nicotine (which is also used as an insecticide) – the part of the cigarette that smokers become addicted to.

3. **Would you give up smoking if you were knowingly going to try for a baby? (This applies to boys too.)**

(Personal response required.)

- Smoking reduces a man's sperm count.
- Even pregnant non-smoking women who have been regularly exposed to passive-smoking tend to have low birth-weight babies, which can also contribute to cot death.
- The chemicals in cigarette smoke reduce the amount of oxygen the baby gets, making the baby's heart beat faster and the baby grow more slowly.

- Spontaneous abortion is more likely, still birth is a third more likely and premature births are twice as likely for pregnant smokers.

4. Should children sue parents or guardians who are responsible for their developing smoking-related illnesses through passive smoking?

(Personal response required.)

(Babies and children are at greater risk, if a parent or guardian smokes, from chest, ear, nose and throat infections, bronchitis and pneumonia, and are more likely to develop breathing problems as adults. Asthma and allergies can be made worse through passive smoking.)

5. If your home is smoky, are there negotiations you can make with the smokers to keep some areas free from smoke, for your health and the health of your pets?

(Personal response required.)

6. Will there come a time when there is an official policy for smoking-related illnesses not to be treated on the NHS (UK National Health Service)?

- Some hospitals have unofficially started to save money in this way, when patients do not agree to give up smoking.

- The NHS regularly features in the news as being over-stretched. In the future it may be decided that smoking-related illnesses are self-inflicted and therefore not deserving of free treatment. However, this takes a very judgemental view of smoking and, of course, some cancers are triggered by passive smoking rather than actually inhaling from the person's own cigarette.

- There might be some need for government compensation to sufferers of smoking-related illnesses since the law allows them to be freely available to people over the age of 16.

7. Is it fair that non-smoking tax-payers foot the bill for self-induced illnesses such as from tobacco smoking? Should the tobacco

companies themselves have to pay? Or should the government use only the amount they gain from taxes on tobacco to treat patients?

(Personal responses required.)

8. **(a) Why do people smoke?**

- Smoking increases your concentration, relieves tension, fatigue and boredom. It can reduce your weight (it suppresses your appetite) and stops you growing.

- Many people start to smoke because their parents or guardians, siblings or friends smoke. If they are susceptible to peer pressure, they will not be able to say 'no'.

- Others smoke because it gives them a certain image. It is a sign of being independent and rebellious. Some think it's 'cool' to smoke.

- Often, after someone has started smoking, the person becomes addicted to it and can't then stop.

(b) Why do people choose not to smoke?

Because they know it:

- damages their health
- interferes with their growth
- is expensive
- is not 'cool' to have an addiction – they prefer to be in control of their bodies, can make up their own minds and not allow others to force them to do something they know is bad for them
- makes them smell bad.

(c) What are the effects of giving up smoking on the body?

Stopping can produce temporary withdrawal symptoms that include:

- craving for cigarettes
- depression
- drowsiness
- fatigue
- inability to concentrate
- insomnia
- irritability

- nausea
- weight gain (because the appetite is no longer dulled and people tend to nibble to distract themselves from thinking about smoking).

Nicotine gum, patches, tablets and lozenges are sold to help relieve the withdrawal symptoms but these have side effects.

9. Should smoking be banned in public and workplaces to avoid 'passive' smoking?

Yes: Passive smoking can irritate the eyes, nose and throat, cause headaches, dizziness and nausea. A person's allergies and asthma can worsen and pregnant women and people suffering from lung, heart or circulatory disease are at greater risk of developing problems.

No: Workplaces can provide smoking areas for those who do smoke to protect those who don't.

10. Should tobacco companies sponsor sports events, thus giving smoking a 'healthy' image?

Probably not – but then who would sponsor the sports? Presumably a company with a healthier image would have been accepted above cigarette manufacturers had they offered.

STORY 31: *The Party*

Tina and her best friend, Seema, were discussing the party Tina had been invited to. Seema was not going as her parents did not allow her out in the evenings.

'I'm so excited about tonight. I've worked out exactly what I'm going to wear,' Tina said.

Seema regarded Tina thoughtfully. Why was this party so special? Tina was always going to parties. 'Is this effort in aid of anyone in particular?'

'Paul. I really fancy Paul! I heard he was going too. I just can't wait, Seema!'

'Isn't he a bit old for you?'

'No. I'm 16, just like his latest ex,' Tina defended herself. Seema was as bad as her parents for not accepting she was grown up.

'Ashish, are you going to that party tonight?' Seema asked.

Ashish nodded. He was glad his little sister wasn't allowed to go. It would cramp his style. 'Why?'

'Oh, I just wondered. You're friends with Paul aren't you? Could you ask him to be nice to Tina – she really fancies him. Don't tell him that though!'

'Does she? Well, well, well.'

Tina arrived half an hour after the party had started and went to the kitchen for a drink. There were soft drinks, beer and cider. David's parents didn't allow spirits, but they did get smuggled in anyway – and his parents weren't to know as they always went next door for the evening.

Paul was standing in the doorway. He smiled and offered to get her a drink. Instead of handing it to her and carrying on with his conversation he suggested they went and danced. Tina was on her way to heaven.

The evening went well, with them chatting on the settee and kissing and cuddling. There was plenty to drink too and Paul had brought his own supply of whisky in his hip flask.

Tina knew she wanted him. She also knew that his previous girlfriends were mostly older than she and more sophisticated. He would expect her to sleep with him. In fact, he'd just asked her to go upstairs for a bit more peace and quiet…

Tina decided it was all right as they were bound to have a long relationship – they just had to as they got on so well. They went up separately, pretending to use the loo and nipping into David's bedroom.

It was dark which was probably why Paul fumbled so much while taking off her clothes. So, this is what sex was all about! A ripple of excitement rushed through Tina's body…

It was over so quickly that Tina barely had time to register what had happened. She didn't feel elated but disgusted. It had been painful and horrible; a few grunts and a gush of sticky fluid running out from her. She felt sick.

On her way out of the toilet, she saw Paul run into his ex and they hugged as if they were still together. Tina felt unutterably stupid.

Four weeks later Tina told her mum she was pregnant. After the initial abusive language, Mrs Posca calmed down. 'It's your decision. It has to be. But let me warn you that I'm not going to bring up the baby for you if you do decide to keep it. I'll help, but the baby's yours. I've done with nappies and colic and I'm finally free to go out more now that you're older. I've got my life too.'

Tina was torn apart. Her religion forbade abortion. But she was still at school!

Discussion Sheet 31: The Party

1. (a) This story has left out the feelings young people have when they are attracted to someone else. How do you feel when you are attracted to someone?

   (b) How do you think a relationship should develop?

   (c) Are there 'stages' you think people should go through that end up with having sex?

2. Why do you think Paul made an immediate play for Tina?

3. (a) Explain as fully as you can why Tina decided to have sex with Paul.

(b) Had she expected the possibility to arise before she'd arrived?

4. (a) What else, apart from the risk of pregnancy, did Tina expose herself to?

(b) How could she have ensured this did not happen?

5. (a) If you were a parent or guardian what stand would you take about a teenage daughter going out?

(b) Would your rules be different for a son of the same age? Why?

6. Why do you think Tina was disappointed with her experience of sex?

7. (a) Was it unfair of Tina's mother to say she was not prepared to look after the baby?

(b) What would you do as a parent or guardian?

(c) Should the issue have been discussed with Tina's dad present?

8. How do you think Paul would have reacted to the pregnancy?

9. How do you think Tina felt about being pregnant with Paul's baby?

10. (a) What would you do in Tina's place? Try to think about her predicament as deeply as you can.

(b) How would your parents or guardians react?

Leader Sheet 31: The Party

1. **(a) *This story has left out the feelings young people have when they are attracted to someone else. How do you feel when you are attracted to someone?***

   - Afraid of being rejected.
   - Excited when you are with the person (sexually and as in really enjoying the person's company).
   - Jealous when you see him or her talking to someone else.
   - Like you're walking on air when you're with him or her.
   - Possessive – you want to be with the person all the time. You want to keep him or her to yourself.
   - Scared that your friends will say something to him or her and that you'll get made fun of.
   - Tense – you have all these pent-up feelings and wonder how he or she feels. You feel anxious and self-conscious when he or she's around.
   - Very alive.
   - Warm and happy when you're with the person.
   - Worried in case he or she doesn't feel the same way.

   (b) *How do you think a relationship should develop?*

   (Personal response required.)

   (This question refers to whether a relationship should develop slowly and lovingly without focusing on sex or whether the person feels that a relationship is not worth having if it doesn't lead to sex fairly quickly.)

   (c) *Are there 'stages' you think people should go through that end up with having sex?*

   (Personal response required.)

   (This question refers to people thinking that they must kiss on their first date, feel a girl's breasts on the third, feel each other's genitals a week later and mutually masturbate for some time after that – and only then move on to sex. It is important for people to realise that they do not have to do this and they do not have to have sex. They can enjoy each other's company and enjoy the pleasures of touching and kissing. It doesn't have to go further.)

2. **Why do you think Paul made an immediate play for Tina?**

Ashish must have told Paul that Tina fancied him so Paul saw her as an easy and willing target for his sexual advances.

3. **(a) Explain as fully as you can why Tina decided to have sex with Paul.**

- Tina was flattered that Paul showed her so much attention.

- Tina knew Paul would probably expect sex once he'd shown an interest in her as he'd had sex with his previous girlfriends.

- Tina wondered what sex was like and perhaps felt it was her turn to find out.

- Tina justified their having sex by convincing herself that it was the start of a long and faithful relationship (despite knowing that Paul had had several exes).

- She had romantic ideas about sex and lovemaking and probably thought that Paul would feel the same.

- She knew that Paul's previous girlfriends were older and more sophisticated than she. Tina wanted to prove to Paul that she was like them, because that was what she thought he wanted.

(b) Had she expected the possibility to arise before she'd arrived?

No – she'd only hoped that Paul would notice her. She didn't imagine he would pay her so much attention, particularly as she was younger and less sophisticated than his usual girlfriends.

4. **(a) What else, apart from the risk of pregnancy, did Tina expose herself to?**

She'd exposed herself to sexually transmitted diseases, most of which are treatable, but one of which is potentially fatal – AIDS. She could have caught HIV, the virus that triggers AIDS.

Other sexually transmitted diseases include:

Candidiasis: caused by a fungus that lives in the vagina and penis. It is also known as thrush. It can spread to

	other warm and moist areas of the body and can live in the sufferer's intestines.
Chlamydia:	can cause infertility. It affects about 10 per cent of teenagers who are sexually active.
Cystitis:	caused by bacteria entering the urinary tract.
Genital herpes:	caused by a virus that produces a sore, blistering and itchy rash. It cannot be cured and attacks recur (like cold sores around the mouth).
Genital warts:	caused by a virus and are linked to increased risk of cervical cancer.
Gonorrhoea:	caused by bacteria. If untreated in women it can cause infection in the Fallopian tubes, which can lead to infertility. (It is also called the clap.)
Pubic lice:	small wingless insects that live in pubic hair and feed on blood.
Scabies:	skin infection caused by a small mite that burrows under the skin to lay eggs. It is highly contagious.
Syphilis:	caused by bacteria that gains access through mucous membranes; the disease can be acquired just by kissing an infected person.
Thrush:	see candidiasis.
Trichomoniasis:	caused by a micro-organism that lives in the vagina and penis.
Viral hepatitis:	affects the person's liver. After diagnosis through a blood test, bed rest, nourishing food and an abstinence of alcohol may help the sufferer recover.

Some of the above infections can be caught without having had sexual intercourse – through kissing or touching an infected person, or through using an infected towel. Sometimes the sufferer becomes infected through organisms in his or her own bowel. Symptoms are not always present so the person does not always know he or she has an infection.

(b) How could she have ensured this did not happen?

- She could have asked Paul to wear a condom. If she had been prepared, she could have taken a condom with her.
- She could have worn a Femidom (the female condom).
- She could have used a diaphragm (or cap) (and used with spermicide it can also protect her against pregnancy).

(All these would prevent HIV being passed to Tina as long as she had no genital sores but other infections can be caught. For example, infective organisms from around her vagina and bowel can be rubbed into her urethra during intercourse causing cystitis. Women prone to cystitis should urinate immediately after sex to flush the urethra.)

Note: If a couple are engaging in oral sex, they can protect themselves by using a dental dam which is a small square of latex to put over the vulva or anus, obtainable from some chemists and sexual health clinics or through mail order. If a couple use sex toys such as a vibrator, they should use a new condom for each partner and for each region with that partner. They should never be used in the anus and then in the vagina without changing the condom as this can spread infection.

5. **(a)** *If you were a parent or guardian, what stand would you take about a teenage daughter going out?*

She might have to:

- be in by a certain time
- let her parents or guardians know where she is
- let her parents or guardians know whom she's with
- understand the risks of sex
- understand the risks of drug-taking
- understand the risks of alcohol abuse
- promise to never go home alone late at night.

Parents and guardians may also want to know more about their daughter's friends and their parents, in the hope that her friends have been brought up similarly to their daughter and that their parents have similar views and restrictions as themselves.

(b) *Would your rules be different for a son of the same age? Why?*

Probably, yes (although the points raised regarding the girls are just as valid for boys).

- Boys are not as likely as girls to be raped or sexually assaulted.
- They don't run the risk of getting pregnant. (But they run the same risks as a girl of having a baby and boys are not usually the ones who get to choose the outcome of a pregnancy.)

- Parents and guardians don't usually feel as protective of their sons as their daughters.

However, boys may be more likely than girls to abuse alcohol or experiment with drugs. They are probably more worried about losing face than a girl so might find it harder to say 'no'.

6. Why do you think Tina was disappointed with her experience of sex?

- It destroyed her romantic view of lovemaking.
- Paul had not bothered to make sex a pleasurable experience for Tina.
- Paul had 'taken' Tina rather than it being a mutual experience on equal terms. He had probably just plunged in, come and rolled off her.
- It had hurt her. This can often happen if the woman is dry or if it's her first time.
- She was disgusted by the actual experience, her fantasies about sex shattered.
- She was disgusted about the mess Paul's semen had made.
- She was probably disgusted at herself once reality had hit.

7. (a) Was it unfair of Tina's mother to say she was not prepared to look after the baby?

Yes: She should support her daughter and help her out. That's what mothers are for.

No: Tina is growing up. By becoming pregnant she'd done a very adult thing and had no right to expect her mother to be tied down for another 16 years just so that Tina could continue to enjoy herself. This decision is Tina's and it has to be hers alone without thinking there is going to be major domestic back-up from her mother.

(b) What would you do as a parent or guardian?

(Personal response required.)

(c) Should the issue have been discussed with Tina's dad present?

Yes:

- Tina's decision could affect the whole family.

- Her dad had a right to know what had happened.

No:

- Many dads get extremely upset about finding out their little girls have become grown-up enough to have sex. He might take out his anger on her.

- To have another critical eye on Tina may have been too much for her. She must have been terribly nervous about telling her mum. If she'd known she'd have to tell both parents together, she may have hidden her pregnancy until it was too late to have a choice or get help.

- It was perhaps better to get her mum's reaction first and deal with that before another person became involved. It made her thoughts and approach more clear-cut without confusing her with masses of emotional feelings and criticisms.

- He may have bullied her to have a termination without letting her make up her own mind, so the family could save face.

Don't know:

- It would depend on who the parents were. Some might take that sort of news better than others.

8. ***How do you think Paul would have reacted to the pregnancy?***

He might:

- be shocked
- deny responsibility
- say he was going to have nothing to do with any baby.

It is reasonable to assume Paul would act negatively, given how he had behaved in the story. He obviously did not care at all for Tina, going straight into an ex-girlfriend's arms after having had sex with Tina. He also hadn't asked Tina about contraception before they had sex, so we know he's irresponsible. We also know he was drunk – he may not even remember having sex with Tina (although if he were that drunk he may have been impotent from the alcohol).

Even if he did acknowledge that the baby could be his, Paul is unlikely to want a lifelong bond of any kind with someone he barely knows. As he seems a bit of a 'lad', he does not appear ready for responsibility, being too interested in girls and drink.

9. How do you think Tina felt about being pregnant with Paul's baby?

- Alone – this problem was hers and inside her. She couldn't just walk away. And none of her friends had been in this situation so she felt she didn't have anyone but her mum to confide in. But even her mum didn't know how she felt.

- Angry that she'd become pregnant by someone as immature and irresponsible as Paul.

- Angry that she'd given her virginity to, and allowed herself to become pregnant by, someone who didn't value her at all.

- Ashamed that everyone would know she'd had sex. And to make it worse, everyone would know it had been a one-night stand, which might make her feel cheap.

- Confused – her previous opinions on life were being challenged. She'd valued her education, but now that was at risk. She was religious and probably previously thought abortion would never be an option for her.

- Mature – the experience had suddenly aged her.

- Regret – that she hadn't waited for someone special to come along before she'd experimented with sex.

- Terrified – she'd suddenly leapt into the adult world and it was scary. This was one mess her mum couldn't pull her out of. (She could only be supportive.)

10. (a) What would you do in Tina's place? Try to think about her predicament as deeply as you can.

You could have the baby because:

- it is a living thing and that has to be considered above all else

- your religion does not allow abortion and you don't feel able to go against your faith because you think you couldn't bear the guilt

- your parents or guardians won't let you have an abortion

- you are thinking of having the baby adopted

- it isn't the baby's fault that you aren't in a stable relationship, independent of parental or guardian care, so why should you take it out on him or her?

You could have an abortion because you:

- are not yet ready to be a mother and are still effectively a child yourself
- don't want anyone to know what has happened
- want to forget that night ever happened and think this is the best way to do it
- are not ready to be in an adult world with adult responsibilities
- want choice in your life and you cannot have that if you tie yourself down at such a young age to having a baby
- know what career you want and you want it desperately. Having a baby would prevent that from ever happening
- don't feel you could be a 'proper mother' anyway.

(b) How would your parents or guardians react?

(Personal response required.)

STORY 32: *Tina's Decision*

When Tina came round from the anaesthetic, she felt an overwhelming sense of relief. She had been so frightened of the consequences of her pregnancy and had wanted to banish all memory of it as soon as possible, before anyone at school could find out. They assumed she had been off with a virus for the past week.

There was no physical pain after the procedure whatsoever. She had a pad between her legs to soak up the mild bleeding. It was just like having a period.

But as she became more awake Tina felt the huge wave of guilt lash out and she knew she had done something seriously contrary to her religion and previous beliefs. She had once privately condemned women who resorted to terminating their pregnancies. She had had such strong ideas on the issue and now they merely mocked her.

At home, all Tina saw were babies on the television, babies in the supermarket, babies and pregnant women everywhere. She felt haunted. What sex would the child have been? What colour hair would her child have had? What colour eyes?

Knowing she couldn't go on like this, Tina visited her older cousin, Sabina.

'Why did you have the termination, Tina?'

'I didn't want a baby. I'm too young. I'm still at school. How could I have provided for it or have been capable of being a good mother? I was terrified. I just wanted to get rid of it. I was ashamed of what people would say.'

'And the father?'

'I didn't tell him.' Tina looked away. 'He had no rights over the baby. It was my body. He would have been horrified. He wouldn't have wanted it. I realised I didn't even like him. I did not want his child and I certainly didn't want him!'

'And how do you feel now?'

'Horrible. Guilty, dirty and a murderess. I'm Catholic but can't face confession. I don't go to church anymore either.'

'Do you regret what you did?' Sabina asked.

'Yes. But I'd do it again if I went back in time. I know I'm not ready to be a mother.'

'Your baby may never have become a baby. And would it have made sense to you to have brought another unwanted child into the world? Would you have resented it? Blamed it for your curtailed life? And you would not have had the support of a loving partner,' Sabina reasoned.

'But I still destroyed something that was living. I don't deserve to have children, ever.'

'Look, you did not destroy something that could live of its own accord. It only had the potential. And you don't know for certain that it would have done. If someone in your class was in the same situation what would you say?'

'Look to the future. Learn from the experience. Make sure that next time she has sex she is well protected against pregnancy, or don't have it at all until she is ready to accept a pregnancy with the help of a loving partner,' Tina stated. She'd had plenty of time to think that through.

'OK. And if her guilt was tied in with her religion?'

'She's paid the price from the misery it's caused. If the priest is going to make her feel worse about herself, leave it until she can take it. Or leave it altogether.'

'It's not easy, Tina. You're just going to have to let time heal. You made a mistake and you need to forgive yourself for it. Grieve for your loss. But get it into perspective – if it wasn't right for you to have the baby, it wasn't right for your baby either.'

Discussion Sheet 32: Tina's Decision

1. There are two forms of contraception available to use after unprotected sex has taken place. What are they, where would you get them from and how soon must you receive treatment if you do not wish to become pregnant?

2. What is the earliest time you can get a pregnancy confirmed?

3. What are your views on abortion? Could it be an option for you or do you feel it would never be acceptable to you? (Assuming you have not yet experienced it.)

4. (a) Did Paul have a right to be told about the pregnancy?

   (b) If your answer is 'no', would it stay the same if Paul and Tina have a close and loving relationship?

5. If Tina had the baby, and did not give him or her up for adoption, what sacrifices would she have to make?

6. What problems does Tina have to face now that she has had the termination?

7. Do you think Tina over-reacted to her feelings of guilt? How would you feel? (Or how have you felt?)

8. (a) Do you agree with the view that no one has a right to pass judgement over another, especially if that person has not yet experienced the particular predicament?

   (b) Do you agree with the view Sabina expressed in the final sentence of the story?

9. (a) What conditions have to be satisfied before a woman can get a legal abortion?

   (b) Why might she choose to have an abortion? (Think of as many reasons as you can.)

10. What are the different types of abortion available? When can these be carried out?

Leader Sheet 32: Tina's Decision

1. *There are two forms of contraception available to use after unprotected sex has taken place. What are they, where would you get them from and how soon must you receive treatment if you do not wish to become pregnant?*

   - The 'morning-after pill'. It consists of two special doses and has to be taken within 72 hours after sex.
   - The IUD (intra-uterine device or coil). This must be fitted within five days after sex.

   Both are available free from doctor's surgeries, Family Planning Clinics and Brook Advisory Centres. If you can't get to these, then a hospital Accident and Emergency department may help. Alternatively, over-16-year-olds can now buy the 'morning-after pill' from pharmacies in the UK at a cost of £20.

2. *What is the earliest time you can get a pregnancy confirmed?*

   You can get a pregnancy confirmed the day your period is due. You can get the test done in your doctor's surgery, but you will have to wait a couple of days for the result. Home pregnancy kits can give an immediate result.

3. *What are your views on abortion? Could it be an option for you or do you feel it would never be acceptable to you? (Assuming you have not yet experienced it.)*

   (Personal response required.)

4. *(a) Did Paul have a right to be told about the pregnancy?*

   Yes: He was the father and he should therefore have rights.

   No: It is Tina's body and it should only be her decision whether she wants to give birth.

   (b) If your answer is 'no', would it stay the same if Paul and Tina have a close and loving relationship?

   Yes: It is still Tina's body and whether or not to carry the pregnancy to full term must still be her decision.

   No: If they are in a stable relationship the father should definitely be told.

5. *If Tina had the baby, and did not give him or her up for adoption, what sacrifices would she have to make?*

- Her education would probably be at an end. It would be possible for her to continue at night school or at college if she had help in looking after her baby. However, this help would have to come from her own parents (if Paul's weren't interested) as she would not have any money to pay for childcare.

- Her chosen career (if she'd had one) may never materialise. It would be extremely hard for her to finish her education and then receive training while having a baby to look after.

- She would have lost the rest of her childhood. She would not be able to go out and have fun without the approval and support of her parents.

- She would not be financially well off (unless supplemented by her parents' money) and would not be likely to earn a significant wage should she be able to find a job that tied in with available childcare as she wouldn't be qualified for specialised work.

- She might find it hard to keep her old friends – their lives would be moving apart, they would have less in common and Tina might resent their freedom.

- She might also find it hard to find a boyfriend. Having a baby would interfere with her freedom to go out and meet people and to sustain an outside relationship. And the boyfriend would need to accept that Tina had commitments that often prevented her from being with him. If the relationship were to look serious, would her boyfriend want to be involved in bringing up another man's child? (Many might, but some might not.)

6. *What problems does Tina have to face now that she has had the termination?*

- She feels horrible, guilty, dirty and a murderess.

- She has to face the fact that she went against the teachings of her faith.

- There is a small possibility she has an infection from the procedure.

- She may become depressed and need counselling.

7. *Do you think Tina over-reacted to her feelings of guilt? How would you feel? (Or how have you felt?)*

(Personal responses required.)

8. (a) *Do you agree with the view that no one has a right to pass judgement over another, especially if that person has not yet experienced the particular predicament?*

(Personal response required.)

(b) *Do you agree with the view Sabina expressed in the final sentence of the story?*

(Personal response required.)

9. (a) *What conditions have to be satisfied before a woman can get a legal abortion?*

To have a legal abortion, two doctors have to agree (under the Abortion Act 1967) that continuing the pregnancy:

- involves a greater risk of injury to the woman's physical or mental health than if the pregnancy were terminated
- involves a greater risk to the woman's life than terminating it
- means that existing children are likely to suffer
- might produce a deformed or seriously handicapped baby.

The woman's financial and social circumstances can also be taken into account if she is less than 24 weeks pregnant.

(b) *Why might she choose to have an abortion? (Think of as many reasons as you can.)*

- She's not in a steady relationship and neither she nor her partner feel ready to take it to the next stage.
- She is still completing her education or training and is not willing to sacrifice her chances of a good career.
- There might be too much else going on in her life to take on an additional burden, such as having a terminally ill relative to care for or her partner being unemployed or her home being repossessed.
- Her partner might have left her or she may have become pregnant through a casual encounter and is not prepared to go it alone and be a single mother.

- Her partner might not want a child and she would risk losing him (or her) if she did have the baby.
- Neither partner wanted children in the first place.
- Her family has already grown up and she does not want to start again. She wants to do something else with her life now.
- She is widowed and does not want to bring up a child on her own.
- She does not have the finances to support a child.
- Her family is complete and she does not feel able to cope with another child.
- Because she has experienced a very bad pregnancy (such as being dangerously ill with high blood pressure or excessive vomiting throughout the nine months) or because she suffered the trauma of her previous baby being stillborn and cannot cope with the possibility of it happening again.
- She is terribly afraid of pregnancy and childbirth, to the extent it has become a phobia. Or she might fear being sick (being emetophobic) and so cannot contemplate 'morning sickness'.
- To save her life – because the pregnancy is causing dangerously high blood pressure or because she has been in an accident and her uterus (womb) has ruptured. Or she might have very poor health and cannot cope with the bodily strain of pregnancy or childbirth.

10. What are the different types of abortion available? When can these be carried out?

Pregnancy is measured in weeks *from the date of the woman's last period.* This means that on the day her period is due, she is already considered to be four weeks pregnant. Women opting for abortion are always offered counselling. It is also available after an abortion if the woman has trouble coming to terms with her feelings.

Menstrual aspiration

This can be performed only up to six or seven weeks from the last menstrual period. This is rarely used as there are too many delays in referring women. A curette (scraper) is used with suction (from a syringe) under local anaesthetic. The cervix does not need to be dilated.

Medical abortion

This is having an abortion without surgery, inducing a miscarriage with drugs. It is available for up to nine weeks of pregnancy. It involves an initial assessment and usually three visits to the hospital or clinic. Mifegyne tablets are taken in the presence of a doctor and you remain at the clinic for two hours afterwards to ensure you do not vomit. Two days later you return to the clinic to have a pessary inserted into the vagina which causes contractions and you remain in the clinic for six hours during which time the abortion usually takes place. You return to the clinic a week or so later so that the doctor can check that all is well. This type of abortion is not suitable for all patients.

Vacuum aspiration or suction

This is the most common method and, if carried out between eight and twelve weeks of pregnancy, it is usually done under local anaesthetic. If the pregnancy is between 13 and 19 weeks, a general anaesthetic is needed as the cervix will need to be dilated first to remove all the contents of the womb.

Prostaglandin or induced abortion

This is for between 19 and 24 weeks of pregnancy and involves a two-night stay and a general anaesthetic. There are five phases – giving medication (prostaglandins) to induce labour, waiting (up to 12 or 18 hours before 'labour' starts), the contractions, the expulsion of the foetus and placenta, and a D and C (under general anaesthetic) to remove any remaining tissue. (D and C is dilation and curettage. The woman's cervex is dilated, or stretched open, and a spoon-shaped curette is used scrape the lining of the uterus to remove any possible placental remains.)

Hysterotomy

This is similar to Caesarian section but is rarely done as risks of complications are much greater. (It might be done, for example, if the woman is allergic to prostaglandins.)

The earlier a woman seeks an abortion, the less risk to her health and the easier it is. For example, an early suction abortion performed under local anaesthetic takes only five minutes. Many abortions are available under the NHS (it depends on where in the UK you live). Many private clinics offer the same treatment without long delays.

STORY 33: No!!

Caroline Summers was on her first date with Andrew Harvey, a boy who had left school last year. She wore new velvet trousers that her mum had treated her to, knowing how much this date meant to her.

They sat in the pub, Andrew with a pint of bitter and Caroline with half a lager.

'What time do you have to be home?' Andrew asked.

'Eleven.' Caroline pulled a face. Her parents were quite strict.

Andrew looked at his watch. 'Shall we go to my place and listen to some CDs? You might like me to tape you some.'

Caroline knew he lived at home with his parents and he had brothers and sisters. 'Yes. That would be good.'

Andrew let them in with his key and put the light on. The rest of the house was in darkness. Caroline knew they were alone.

'My CD player's in my room. Second on the right,' Andrew told her after taking her coat and hanging it up.

'OK.' Caroline smiled weakly. He'd think her a real child if she made a fuss. She climbed the stairs.

'What would you like on first?' Andrew asked as they got in the room. It was spacious with a desk, chair, single bed and lots of shelves and a wardrobe. 'How about that sixties CD I was telling you about?'

'Fine.' Caroline wondered where to sit.

'Relax.' Andrew smiled. 'Come and sit down.' He led her to the bed and sat her down next to him, holding her hand.

They talked for about half an hour before Andrew leant over to kiss her. It was wonderful. After her initial shyness, she responded to him. But soon he eased down and lay half on top of her. She felt nervous. Then he started to undress her. Caroline tried to sit up. This was too quick for her.

'Hey, you know you're enjoying this just as much as I am. Let yourself go. There's no need to feel guilty,' Andrew murmured.

But Caroline wasn't happy. She wanted to sit up again. Andrew held her down, kissing her frantically. He fiddled with his jeans and then pushed his hand down the soft waistband of her trousers.

'No!!' Caroline realised with a shock what it was he wanted to do. She struggled and tried to kick but his weight was on her and one of his hands held hers while the other was tugging at her trousers…

When it was over Andrew rolled off. 'Well, admit it. You enjoyed it. You wanted it too.'

'Where's the bathroom?' Caroline whispered.

She didn't wait to be told but ran until she found it, holding on to her clothes. She was immediately sick in the toilet and sat on the floor shaking. She had to get away. And her parents must never know. They would think her cheap. They would say she had led him on, that it was her fault.

When Caroline got in, she went into her mum's bedroom to tell her she was home.

'Did you have a nice time, dear?' her mother asked sleepily.

'Great. It was great. Thanks Mum.' Caroline turned to leave. 'Oh, I'm just going to take a shower. Someone knocked drink all over me.' She felt violated and used and doubted she'd ever feel clean. She would make sure her trousers were stained so badly she could never wear them. And she would never ever trust any man again.

Discussion Sheet 33: No!!

1. (a) Why had Caroline thought she would be safe at Andrew's house?

    (b) Could Caroline have foreseen what was going to happen? Give reasons.

2. For Caroline, it wasn't safe to go to Andrew's house on her first date. How long would you (if you are a girl) leave it before going to your boyfriend's place? Do you trust easily?

3. Andrew did not accept Caroline's 'No!!' Some men, including Andrew, interpret a woman's 'no' as a 'yes'. Have you experienced this (if you are a girl)? Have you done this yourself (if you are a boy)?

4. The type of rape Caroline experienced is known as 'date rape'. It is hard to prove. Why do you think this is?

5. (a) Have you ever, in any way, thought that a rape victim must 'have been asking for it'?

   (b) Does it make a difference to your answer if the woman was wearing revealing, 'sexy' clothes?

6. If you want to report a rape to the police, you must do it as soon after the event as you can, before having a shower and without changing your clothes. Why is this?

7. (a) What reaction would your parents or guardians have if you were raped (girls) or if you were accused of rape (boys)?

   (b) How would your parents or guardians react if you were a boy who had been raped?

8. (a) Other than the police, where can you go for help following a rape?

   (b) If you do not want to risk a pregnancy resulting from rape where can you go and how long after the event?

   (c) Where can you go to be checked out for sexually transmitted diseases?

9. (a) How can women and girls reduce the possibilities of being raped?

   (b) How would you feel if you'd been raped (girls) or buggered without consent (boys and girls)?

10. (a) Drug rape is now becoming common. What is it?

    (b) Why does it make rape more difficult to prove?

    (c) How could you protect yourself from drug rape?

Leader Sheet 33: No!!

1. **(a) Why had Caroline thought she would be safe at Andrew's house?**

When he'd asked her back to his house she thought his parents and siblings would be at home.

(b) Could Caroline have foreseen what was going to happen? Give reasons.

No – she'd trusted him. When she arrived and found the house in darkness, although she was scared she still trusted him. It wasn't until he'd started the heavy petting and tugging at her clothes that she realised what he really wanted.

2. **For Caroline, it wasn't safe to go to Andrew's house on her first date. How long would you (if you are a girl) leave it before going to your boyfriend's place? Do you trust easily?**

(Personal responses required.)

3. **Andrew did not accept Caroline's 'No!!' Some men, including Andrew, interpret a woman's 'no' as a 'yes'. Have you experienced this (if you are a girl)? Have you done this yourself (if you are a boy)?**

(Personal responses required.)

4. **The type of rape Caroline experienced is known as 'date rape'. It is hard to prove. Why do you think this is?**

Because she had arranged to meet Andrew and had willingly gone to his home – it is his word against hers that she had not consented to sex. Police might suspect that she's saying that she was raped to cause trouble or because she was frightened of getting into trouble from her parents should she later discover she was pregnant. Unless there is overwhelming evidence to support her claim (such as a trashed room and torn clothes to indicate a struggle) it would be a hard case to prove and virtually impossible if she was not a virgin prior to the rape – past sexual experiences and gynaecological history are used in court to undermine the person's credibility. (The women most protected by the law are virgin daughters and faithful wives.)

5. **(a) *Have you ever, in any way, thought that a rape victim must 'have been asking for it'?***

(Personal response required.)

(b) *Does it make a difference to your answer if the woman was wearing revealing, 'sexy' clothes?*

No woman asks to be raped or sexually assaulted. If she wears revealing clothes that is how she chooses to present herself and her appearance represents part of her personality. Men use the excuse that the woman was 'asking for it' to justify their behaviour. Even if the woman is a prostitute by profession, she still has the right only to have sex with whom she wants under the terms she gives.

6. **If you want to report a rape to the police, you must do it as soon after the event as you can, before having a shower and without changing your clothes. Why is this?**

- Police assume that if you really have been raped you will report it immediately. (However, if you tell a friend about it instead, his or her evidence can be used to testify to what you said and as to your state – for example, if you were dishevelled and shaking with shock.)

- Delay in officially reporting the crime lessens the chance of forensic evidence being found and damages your credibility. (The police may decide to take the matter no further.)

- You mustn't shower or wash before going to the police because it destroys forensic evidence. (You will have a full medical examination after the police have taken your statement.)

7. **(a) *What reaction would your parents or guardians have if you were raped (girls) or if you were accused of rape (boys)?***

Girls: They might be shocked, blaming, accusing, sympathetic, angry at whoever had done this, supportive. They might take charge and organise everything – the police, the medical assistance. They might call you a whore.

Boys: They might be disgusted, shocked, disbelieving, horror-struck, angry that you'd got caught.

(b) How would your parents or guardians react if you were a boy who had been raped?

They might be supportive, or might accuse you of being gay.

8. ### (a) Other than the police, where can you go for help following a rape?

A trusted friend or adult or The Rape Crisis Centre (in the UK). (*Note:* if the crime is reported to the police, it is out of the person's hands as to whether prosecution goes ahead. Rape is an offence against the state – it is the state that decides whether to go ahead with the prosecution and how it will be done. Once rape is reported, it is not easy for the charges to be withdrawn later if the person decides he or she cannot face appearing in court.)

(b) If you do not want to risk a pregnancy resulting from rape where can you go and how long after the event?

You can go to a Family Planning Clinic, your doctor, a hospital's Accident and Emergency department, a Brook Advisory Centre or the British Pregnancy Advisory Service. Or, if you don't mind paying for it, you can go to a pharmacy. The 'morning-after pill' is now available over the counter in the UK for a fee of £20.

You must go within two to five days after sexual intercourse – the earlier the better. The 'morning-after pill' can be given within 72 hours and the IUD (intra-uterine device) fitted within 5 days of sexual intercourse.

(c) Where can you go to be checked out for sexually transmitted diseases?

You will need to go to a STD (sexually transmitted diseases) clinic. The medical examination you get at the police station is only to obtain forensic evidence.

9. ### (a) How can women and girls reduce the possibilities of being raped?

- Don't be out alone late at night. But if you must, keep to well-lit and busy streets if you can. Carry a personal alarm in your pocket.

You could carry an aerosol to aim at the man's eyes (to give you time to run away), but not anything that could be classed as an offensive weapon. Be prepared to run or to enter a busy pub or shop if you feel at risk.

- Don't walk in lonely areas on your own.
- If you've been to a party – or are going to one – cover up sexy clothes with a long unrevealing coat. (To avoid being thought of as provocative and to attract as little unwanted attention as possible.) If necessary, change when you get to the party and again before you go home.
- Don't go into another man's home before you are very sure of him – and don't let him into yours. (Although this is not foolproof – sometimes it is the man you trust.)

Although this advice is aimed at women, it is not to criticise women for attracting trouble – full responsibility lies with men who cannot control themselves or have no wish to do so. Whatever a woman does she can never prevent rape altogether and is not responsible for being raped. There is never an excuse for rape.

(b) How would you feel if you'd been raped (girls) or buggered without consent (boys and girls)?

Note: Rape is penetration of the penis into the vagina or labia (without ejaculation necessarily taking place) without the woman's consent. Buggery is penetration of the anus by a penis.

Girls: Angry, ashamed, depressed, dirty, guilty, powerless, scared, shocked, unclean, vulnerable, unable to cope with what's happened.

Boys: They may also experience the same feelings as mentioned above.

(Boys tend to feel far more shame than girls because it dents their idea of manhood to have been overcome by another man and be so used. Very few men report rape because of their shame and they are less likely to seek counselling so suffer more in silence.)

Rape can deeply affect people for years. It can interfere with their future and current relationships and can make victims lose trust in people. Girls and women might find it impossible to have a sexual relationship with anyone again, feeling repulsion at physical contact. People who have been raped may have terrifying nightmares.

10. (a) Drug rape is now becoming common. What is it?

A person is either given a spiked drink (with a very sedative drug) or the man spikes it while the person goes to the toilet. It can be any drink (tea, coffee, milk, cola) as the drugs are tasteless and odourless. (Although the best-known drug does have a blue dye in it, it does not show for 20 minutes and will not show up in dark drinks anyway.) The man may be someone the person works with – such as at an office party – or a complete stranger. When the person feels nauseous, very tired and odd, the man offers to take him or her home – to outsiders it looks as though the person is drunk. (Many victims are taken back to their own home and raped in their own beds.) Sometimes the person is raped by more than one man – he or she can also be video-taped in the act.

(b) Why does it make rape more difficult to prove?

The person may not realise he or she's been raped until flashbacks tell him or her that something has happened (the drugs used take away the person's memory). The drug may be traced in the body by forensics for two to three days after it was taken. But by the time the person realises what has happened, he or she may have washed away any evidence of sexual intercourse and it might be too late for the drug to be detected.

(c) How could you protect yourself from drug rape?

- Never leave your drink unattended and then go back to it. Either take it with you or discard it and get another.

- Buy your own drinks or watch the person buying it for you very carefully.

- Order canned drinks that you open yourself.

- If you suddenly feel strange, go to someone for help such as the landlord of the pub, and explain what you think has happened. Ask for protection. (He or she may give you a room to sleep it off in, safe from harm, and could call a friend or relative for you if you give the relevant number.)

STORY 34: TO LEAD BAGGY?

My name is Michael and I'm different to others in my class. I don't look any different; I just feel different. Since before my teens. There seems to be some sort of pack instinct whenever I'm around as all the boys go for me. They go in for the kill if they see me out of school or on my own in the schoolyard.

And that happens much more now, as others don't want to be seen with me – because if they are, they get called names too. But not for long. The name-calling stops as soon as they've dropped me.

I am human but I have to remind myself of that since I'm mostly treated like an animal at school, at the receiving end of everyone's jokes and avoided as though I had some nasty disease. The girls snigger behind my back and are just as bad as the boys except they don't physically threaten me.

My home life's not great either. My parents wonder why I don't bring anyone home any more and why I never have a friend phone me up. They're very worried. At least, Mum is. Dad suspects I get picked on and he keeps saying why don't I fight back?

I don't because I'm gentle, I don't like getting hurt and I don't want to hurt anyone else but if nothing changes I expect one day it will all get too much for me. Then I will strike.

I feel very confused and alone. I can't talk to anyone about anything that matters. I'm frightened about what is happening to me and it makes it so much worse that I am hated because I am different. Well, I hate being different too but there's nothing I can do to change the way I am.

I haven't told you about my problem yet because I thought you might stop listening to me before I finished what I want to say. You know, I didn't ask to be like I am. I know I have to make the best of things because I only have one life, according to my religion (which also seems to reject people like me totally unless we lead a life struggling against our natures).

But until people's attitudes change and some dreadful myths are exploded I can see no way forward. How can things change when people don't listen? When they don't *want* to listen?

This is my crime, why I'm a social outcast and should be hidden from family and friends. I prefer men to women. It's true, I do. But this is a homophobic society that we live in where men feel threatened by other men not acting as men 'should'. It is an age of machoism where you have to prove just how good you are at bonking women. Even beating them up won't come amiss with some of the men.

But I'm not like that. I am warm and sensitive and am very easily hurt by the things people say. I pretend that I'm not affected by words such as 'bum boy' and 'fairy', 'woofter' and 'queer'. I pretend that I'm loved for myself alone and not hated because I'm attracted to other men. I pretend I get approval for the things I can do, not disapproval or scorn because I'm attracted to other men. I pretend lots of things but none are true.

Discussion Sheet 34: TO LEAD BAGGY?

1. (a) What does 'homophobic' mean?

    (b) Is Michael right? Try to support your answer with examples.

2. What are your parents' or guardians' views on homosexuality? Do your views mirror these? If they do, can you say that they really are what you yourself believe in, regardless of your parents' or guardians' viewpoint, or is it because you have been influenced by them?

3. What are your friends' views on homosexuality?

4. How would your family and friends react if you were to announce that you were homosexual? Is their love for you complete, regardless of your sexual tendencies, or is it a conditional love that is only there if you conform to the majority?

5. If a homosexual feels unable to 'come out' and decides to conform against his or her natural sexual tendency and marries, explain what you think may happen.

6. (a) What myths about homosexuality do you know? Are they true?

    (b) What stereotypes of gay men have been used in the story?

    (c) Are all gay men like this?

7. (a) Have you ever deliberately picked on someone because you suspect or know that they are homosexual? If so, why?

    (b) Have you ever been picked on for anything at all?

    (c) If so, how did it feel?

8. (a) Do you feel that people should be able to live their private lives as they wish?

    (b) Do you have strong feelings about other people's sexual preferences? If so, why?

9. (a) Have you 'come out' or do you know of someone who has? What was it like for you or for them?

    (b) How would you react to your best friend confiding that he or she is homosexual?

10. What is the title an anagram of?

Leader Sheet 34: TO LEAD BAGGY?

1. **(a) What does 'homophobic' mean?**

   Homophobic means a person has a fear of homosexuality or has a very negative attitude towards it.

   (People with negative attitudes to homosexuals are more likely to have friends with negative attitudes, more likely to be older and less well-educated, more likely to be religious, more conservative and more authoritarian and are more likely to have traditional stereotypical ideas about male and female behaviour.)

   (b) Is Michael right? Try to support your answer with examples.

   Gay people were less tolerated then heterosexuals, particularly if they behaved outside their stereotypes, but this is changing. Negative views on homosexuality may still pervade the older generations and more isolated communities. But as society is more aware of homosexuality and more and more homosexuals 'come out', the less negative interest homosexuality receives. It is only with the less well-educated and uninformed that out-dated opinions still hold.

2. **What are your parents' or guardians' views on homosexuality? Do your views mirror these? If they do, can you say that they really are what you yourself believe in, regardless of your parents' or guardians' viewpoint, or is it because you have been influenced by them?**

   (Personal responses required.)

3. **What are your friends' views on homosexuality?**

   (Personal response required.)

4. **How would your family and friends react if you were to announce that you were homosexual? Is their love for you complete, regardless of your sexual tendencies, or is it a conditional love that is only there if you conform to the majority?**

   (Personal responses required.)

5. **If a homosexual feels unable to 'come out' and decides to conform against his or her natural sexual tendency and marries, explain what you think may happen.**

('Coming out' is when gays or lesbians identify themselves as such publicly.)

The person may have extra-marital affairs with those of the same sex or leave the heterosexual relationship altogether for a homosexual one. (Many women who have been married and have had children later decide that they want a lesbian relationship.) It can cause more distress to both sides than being honest in the first place.

6. **(a) What myths about homosexuality do you know? Are they true?**

- Homosexuals fancy everyone the same sex as themselves. (This is not true – their tastes vary as do heterosexuals'.)

- Lesbians are man-haters and gay men fear women. (This is not true – homosexuals have friends of either sex as do heterosexuals.)

- Women who aren't attractive to men become lesbians. (This is not true – women are lesbians because that is how they are, not because they can't 'get a man'.)

- You can recognise a homosexual by the way he or she behaves, dresses or talks. (This is not true. Not all butch women are lesbians and not all lesbians look butch and have short hair. Not all effeminate men are gay nor are all gay men effeminate, wearing extrovert and brightly coloured clothes.)

- Homosexuals wish they were the opposite sex. (This is not true. They do not want a sex change, they are happy being the sex they are.)

- Gay men are promiscuous. (Some are, some aren't, just as with heterosexuals.)

- Gay men are paedophiles. (Some are, most aren't, just as with heterosexuals.)

(b) What stereotypes of gay men have been used in the story?

- Michael is portrayed as a victim, unable to stand up for himself.
- He is emotionally sensitive.
- He is gentle.

(c) Are all gay men like this?

No. Gay men have the same traits as non-gay men.

7. (a) Have you ever deliberately picked on someone because you suspect or know that they are homosexual? If so, why?

(Personal responses required.)

(b) Have you ever been picked on for anything at all?

(Personal response required.)

(c) If so, how did it feel?

You might feel: angry, scared, shamed, small, useless and vulnerable.

8. (a) Do you feel that people should be able to live their private lives as they wish?

Yes, as long as their behaviour does not harm anyone or negatively affect others' lives.

(b) Do you have strong feelings about other people's sexual preferences? If so, why?

(Personal responses required.)

9. (a) Have you 'come out' or do you know of someone who has? What was it like for you or for them?

(Personal responses required.)

(b) How would you react to your best friend confiding that he or she is homosexual?

Ideally with open curiosity so that your interested questions lead to understanding. And ideally you would also be non-judgemental and supportive.

10. What is the title an anagram of?

'Glad to be gay?'

STORY 35: *Perspective*

Dear Mum and Dad,

Please read this letter together, at the same time! Are you BOTH there? Now please sit down.

As you know, my exam results were due to come this morning – but actually, they were in yesterday's post. I didn't tell you because I had a lot on my mind and needed to sort things out, to decide what to do. Well, now I have. You needn't worry about my grades as they were all As and Bs. But I'm not going any further with my education.

I'm sorry this will be such a shock to you as I know you had great plans for me. But I also know how much you are looking forward to being grandparents. And soon you will be. As you read this, I'll be sitting on a train to Brighton, going to a home for unmarried mothers. I was given the address by this kind lady at the Samaritans. The baby is due in December. Maybe I'll call you after you've had time to get used to the idea and then I can come home to have the baby?

No, the father hasn't left me but at the moment, he's not in a position to help. He's a very kind and well-meaning person but not very well-educated. However, his reading is coming along just fine since I started to give him lessons. It was such a shame that he was set up by someone who asked him to do a favour and is now doing a short stretch for aiding and abetting a robbery of a building society. He's had such bad luck since leaving school, including employment. I'm told it gets harder once you've reached 30.

Yes, he is quite a bit older than I am but he's very young at heart and great fun to be with. He's quite responsible in many ways, too. He made sure he got his infection cleared up as soon as he knew there was a problem and made sure I had a check too in case the baby got harmed. But we've both been treated for it now and are fine.

He comes from a well-respected family. His grandfather was quite high up in the Mafia in Sicily before his liver gave out. When his father was executed his mother came to Britain but she does find it hard to cope on her own in a foreign country and so is helped with anti-depressants. She's had a hard life.

I know you do not really approve of cross-culture and cross-religion marriage but I'm sure you'll like Marcus when he's released from prison. We are hoping that as you've got such a big house we would be able to start our married life with you. You'll soon get used to the baby not being pure black – it will be exciting to find out just what shade he or she will be. Marcus has such a generous nature that I'm sure you'll quickly see beyond the white of his skin just as I did.

Now that I've told you all that, I want to tell you that I am not pregnant, I am not going to Brighton, there is no Marcus, I had no venereal disease and I am not involved with any man at present. But I didn't get As and Bs. The highest grade was a D. I just wanted you to see the marks in the proper perspective. I'll be back for lunch.

Your loving daughter,

Esmé

Author's note: *This letter was inspired by another letter, read out on radio by Alistair Cooke. It was written from the College of Fine Arts, Albany, New York, July 3, 1967.*

Discussion Sheet 35: Perspective

1. (a) Do you feel your parents or guardians need a lesson in 'perspective'?

   (b) What approach could you use? (Don't copy Esmé's idea, as it may cause great distress.)

2. (a) What were Esmé's parents' expectations of their daughter?

   (b) What are your own expectations of yourself? Are they in perspective?

3. (a) Do you push yourself too hard?

   (b) How would you know? (What are the signs of stress?)

   (c) What can you do to combat stress and exam stress?

4. (a) Do you agree that it doesn't matter what you achieve in life as long as you try your best at everything that comes your way?

   (b) Do you feel it is wrong not to develop any 'talents' that you may have?

5. (a) Do your parents or guardians or your teachers ever compare you unfavourably with an older brother or sister or other person?

   (b) If so, how do you feel about this?

6. It is now well-known that if you tell a child he or she is stupid (or make some other negative comment), the child often fulfils that low expectation. Do your parents or guardians have low expectations of you or none at all? How do you feel about this?

7. Exam results and qualifications are only a small part of you as a person. If you do not cause your parents or guardians any worries (such as with drug abuse, stealing, teenage pregnancy etc.) do you think they should be happy with you?

8. (a) Do you ever worry about something to the extent that the event is seen out of proportion to reality?

   (b) If you do, how can you try to see it in perspective?

9. Does your self-esteem (how you see yourself) depend on how your parents or guardians see you and treat you or are you self-confident and do not need to rely on others for approval?

10. (a) What problems might you have if your self-esteem is low?

    (b) How can you raise your self-esteem?

Leader Sheet 35: Perspective

1. **(a) Do you feel your parents or guardians need a lesson in 'perspective'?**

    (Personal response required.)

    (b) What approach could you use? (Don't copy Esmé's idea, as it may cause great distress.)

    Point out to them that they complain about your behaviour (or exam results) a great deal. Ask them, for example, to be glad that you:

    - come in when they ask
    - do not get drunk
    - do not swear at them
    - have never taken drugs
    - don't smoke
    - are careful with your sexual partners.

    (Obviously, it is up to the individual to choose what comparisons he or she wishes to make. Not all may be relevant for any one person.)

2. **(a) What were Esmé's parents' expectations of their daughter?**

    They wanted her to:

    - do well in her exams and go to university so that she would have a good career
    - marry a black man of the same religion as theirs and from a similar background to their own
    - have children, but not yet.

    (b) What are your own expectations of yourself? Are they in perspective?

    (Personal responses required.)

3. **(a) Do you push yourself too hard?**

    (Personal responses required.)

(b) How would you know? (What are the signs of stress?)

- Abdominal pain.
- Biting nails or picking fingers.
- Diarrhoea.
- Eating more or less than usual.
- Feeling unable to cope.
- Headaches.
- Insomnia.
- Panic attacks and phobias.
- Skin problems. (More acne than usual, eczema and psoriasis.)
- Tense muscles.

(c) What can you do to combat stress and exam stress?

- Be kind to yourself and do not label yourself as a failure for one mistake.
- Ensure you give yourself time to relax and be by yourself.
- Get plenty of exercise – it combats stress and helps you sleep.
- Keep to a routine – this is less stressful than working later than normal and waking up exhausted.
- Learn to relax. (Borrow or buy a book on stress and a relaxation tape.)
- Listen to your mind and body. When you need a break, give yourself one.
- Pace yourself. Don't drive yourself too hard or overload your schedule.
- Treat yourself to something nice every day.
- To combat exam stress, make a realistic revision timetable and stick to it. Timetable in leisure, rest and exercise periods so that you pace yourself. No one can effectively concentrate, for example, eight hours at a stretch without a break.

4. **(a) Do you agree that it doesn't matter what you achieve in life as long as you try your best at everything that comes your way?**

Yes: No one can ask more. If your achievement is lower than someone else's, you should not be made to feel ashamed or worthless. You must learn to accept your limitations and not let them label you as a failure.

No: Your best is not always good enough. When you try hard but still don't succeed, or get the job you want, you feel useless.

(b) Do you feel it is wrong not to develop any 'talents' that you may have?

It is rather a waste of your potential – and you never know when your situation might change and you could make good use of them. For example, you may not bother to do well at school because you have known for years that you will join the family business. This may be, for example, in farming, manufacturing or retailing. But market conditions may change or something else unforeseen may get in the way, such as BSE and foot and mouth disease affecting farmers' livelihoods. You can no longer guarantee that you will be securely employed by a member of your family for the rest of your life. Believing so and acting on the assumption is a big risk to take.

Also, if you do not develop your talents or make the most of yourself, your self-esteem may suffer. You may also find you lack confidence when you are older as you see that others are more capable than you – yet you know you've got the ability within you. Others will not look upon you with respect if they perceive you as lazy or taking short cuts.

5. **(a) Do your parents or guardians or your teachers ever compare you unfavourably with an older brother or sister or other person?**

(Personal responses required.)

(b) If so, how do you feel about this?

That it's unfair:

- You are an individual and want to be seen as such.
- You should not be compared to anyone else and should be recognised in your own right.

- Why should anyone expect you to be similar to a previous pupil from the same family when you are not the same?

(The same can happen when an older sibling has proved to be a challenging pupil – teachers may be wary of the next child from the same family and be too ready to apportion blame and punishment for a misdemeanour that a normally well-behaved child might have got away with relatively lightly.)

6. *It is now well-known that if you tell a child he or she is stupid (or make some other negative comment), the child often fulfils that low expectation. Do your parents or guardians have low expectations of you or none at all? How do you feel about this?*

(Personal responses required.)

7. *Exam results and qualifications are only a small part of you as a person. If you do not cause your parents or guardians any worries (such as with drug abuse, stealing, teenage pregnancy etc.) do you think they should be happy with you?*

(Personal response required.)

8. *(a) Do you ever worry about something to the extent that the event is seen out of proportion to reality?*

(Personal response required.)

(b) If you do, how can you try to see it in perspective?

Tell yourself:

- It's not the end of the world. Worse things can happen.
- Everyone makes mistakes, it's part of human nature.
- You can use the experience and learn from it – you'll know better next time.
- One mistake does not make you a failure.
- You are still loved and others will still see your positive attributes.
- If it doesn't work the first time, you can try again. And again.

9. *Does your self-esteem (how you see yourself) depend on how your parents or guardians see you and treat you or are you self-confident and do not need to rely on others for approval?*

(Personal response required.)

10. (a) *What problems might you have if your self-esteem is low?*

You might:

- think so little of yourself that you feel life is not worth living. You may become depressed or even suicidal
- over- or under-eat or develop an eating disorder
- feel tired and need more sleep than usual, or be reluctant to get out of bed in the mornings
- show your distress by having panic attacks or developing phobias, truanting, becoming involved in substance abuse and criminal acts.

Generally, if you have poor self-esteem you are at risk of poor mental health.

(b) *How can you raise your self-esteem?*

- By reminding yourself of all your positive attributes – what you can do and are good at, what people like about you, the number of friends you have – or the fact that with the few friends you do have you have a very good relationship.
- By telling yourself that not everyone can be the same, having different strengths and weaknesses.
- By rewarding yourself for things done well or for any successes, however minor.
- By reassuring yourself that as long as your life is moving forward in some way, you're doing fine. You do not have to measure yourself against others to feel good. You should only be compared with how you were and how you are now.
- By reminding yourself you are an individual with rights (see below) and needs like everyone else. Tell others what your needs are so that they can be recognised.

- Exercise your rights. If someone has done something to upset you or is taking advantage of you, let the person know. And refuse to be further taken advantage of.
- Learn to be assertive to protect yourself and your rights.
- Ban negative images you have of yourself. Think only positive thoughts.
- By treating yourself for no particular reason – just because you are you and so deserve it.

Personal rights:

1. I have the right to express my feelings and opinions.

2. I have the right to say 'no'.

3. I have the right to make mistakes and cope with the consequences.

4. I have the right to change my mind.

5. I have the right to success.

6. I have the right to ask for what I want and to make my needs known.

7. I have the right to be treated with respect.

8. I have the right to refuse responsibility for other people's problems.

Section 4

Introduction

Section 4 is concerned with issues relevant to 16- to 18-year-olds, although it can be used with younger people if there is a need for it. Stories 38 and 39 are interconnected with a developing theme and should be read in order. The rest of the stories in Section 4 can be read in any order.

Section 4 is largely concerned with emotions and relationships. Story 39 is much longer than the others to allow a deeper insight into Trudy's life and the changing relationship between her and her husband, and her and her mother. Story 40 addresses the serious topic of teenage suicide and the questions posed are more demanding than elsewhere in the book so may take longer than one hour to answer, depending on the interest and ability of the individuals.

Summary of Contents

Story/Task	Title	Subject
36	Next Time?	Genetic illnesses, bereavement
	Exercise: Bereavement	Bereavement
37	Escape!	Controlling relationships
	Exercise: Decision-Making – Ending a Relationship	Decision-making in a relationship
38	Marriage*	Marriage, relationships
39	Trudy's Baby*	Teenage motherhood
40	The Last Straw	Teenage suicide

* These stories are interconnected and should be read in order.

STORY 36: *Next Time?*

Heidi still felt a bit weak on her first day back at school after the holiday. She'd spent the first part of the break in hospital having an exchange blood transfusion, as she had not responded to the antibiotics, fluids and oxygen she had been given.

Her mum had wanted her to stay at home for longer but Heidi wanted to get back to the normality of school life and her friends. It was what helped keep her going.

All her life, as far back as she could remember, she had thrown herself into her schoolwork, projects and outings. She was always on the lookout for fun and distractions, knowing she had little time to live her life to the full. It seemed to help her parents too, who had looked at her so proudly while she shouldered the knowledge of her illness as though she wasn't going to let it stand in her way. She was a fighter and always had been. But now her determination had been sapped from her as surely as though it had been sucked out of her in that exchange transfusion.

'Are you OK?' Dara asked, noticing that Heidi was unusually quiet.

Heidi smiled. 'Yeah. I'm OK.'

Dara was doubtful about Heidi's answer and sat down next to her on the bench in the schoolyard. School hadn't yet started. 'Did you have a good holiday?'

Heidi shook her head.

'Neither did I. I had to take on all the housework and cooking so that Mum could do more hours. We needed the money. What was wrong with yours?'

'I wasn't well. I'd caught some kind of infection and my body couldn't cope. I had new blood, which helped. But there'll always be a next time.'

Dara gave Heidi a hug. She wanted to understand but she didn't know enough about sickle cell anaemia. 'Don't feel you have to bottle up your feelings – it's meant to help, talking about problems.'

Heidi sighed. 'I don't like to. It's my problem.'

'But friends are there to help. One day I'll tell you all my problems to make us quits. What's bugging you? You've had crises before and you've never reacted like this – normally you bounce back and are as cheerful as ever. What's different about it now?'

Heidi looked at Dara full on. 'Remember my sister, Natasha, got married last year? Well, she's going to have a baby. That's probably never going to happen to me even if I were to find a partner.

'I know some women have managed to have babies successfully through having regular exchange transfusions to keep them and their baby healthy. But that won't happen to me.

'It seems unfair that Natasha has escaped even being a carrier – I don't wish her ill but I do get jealous and think, why can't I do the things other people take for granted?

'Each time I have a crisis it gets more serious with more damage to my body. The doctors looked surprised when I pulled through and I knew what they thought – that next time might be the last. That's what I think when I'm lying there. About the next time.

'I'm scared, Dara. More scared than I've ever been. Scared of dying, scared of more pain, scared of the loneliness as I lie helpless in bed. I want to live and I know I'm not going to. I want the life other people have and I'm so angry that it's being denied me. It's so *unfair*!'

Dara silently put her arms around Heidi and held her close. Life *was* unfair.

Discussion Sheet 36: Next Time?

1. (a) Heidi has sickle cell anaemia which is a genetically linked disease. What do you understand by this term?

   (b) Can you name other genetically linked diseases?

2. Are any of these linked to racial groups?

3. Are any of them linked to the sex of the person?

4. Do you know of anyone with a terminal illness or who had a terminal illness? If so, what was it?

5. How would you feel if you knew you wouldn't survive past your 20s, and possibly not even as long as that?

6. (a) Are there any genetically linked illnessses in your family?

   (b) If so, you may need to go for genetic counselling before starting a family of your own. Why is that?

7. If you and your partner were both carrying a serious genetically linked disease, do you think that you would go ahead with starting a family? (With genetically linked diseases, if both partners are carriers, there is a 25 per cent – 1 in 4 – chance of passing the full disease on to their offspring and another 50 per cent – 1 in 2 – chance of making their offspring carriers of the disease. So there is a 25 per cent chance of having a completely healthy baby.)

8. If one of your friends had a serious illness, how would you support him or her?

9. Why is it especially hard for parents, guardians and friends to cope with death in a young person?

10. (a) Have you experienced bereavement?

    (b) If so, how did you feel?

    (c) How would you like to have been supported through your grief?

Leader Sheet 36: Next Time?

1. **(a) Heidi has sickle cell anaemia, which is a genetically linked disease. What do you understand by this term?**

   Genetically linked diseases are caused wholly or partly by a fault in the person's genes, which are the blueprints for that person's body. When genetic material is faulty, abnormal proteins can be made causing disturbances in body chemistry that lead to disease. The genetic fault may occur only in certain races or in certain sexes and in these instances, the resulting disease is called a racially linked or sex linked disorder.

   (Sickle cell anaemia is a racially linked illness that is very common in black people and less so in Mediterranean people. The sufferer's red blood cells contain abnormal haemoglobin, which results in a very severe form of anaemia. The blood cells are distorted and very fragile. Sickle cells offer some resistance to the parasite causing malaria that reproduces in normal blood cells – this is an example of how races have adapted to cope with malaria – but the sickle cells have less capacity for carrying oxygen. Out of malarial areas, the sickle cell cannot be viewed as a positive trait as it only poses a liability and is carried on through the genes from one generation to the next.)

   (b) Can you name other genetically linked diseases?

   Other genetically linked diseases (found in both sexes) are:

Albinism	This is a lack of the pigment melanin that gives colour to skin, hair and eyes, and it occurs in all races.
Down syndrome	This is due to a chromosomal abnormality resulting in mental impairment and a characteristic physical appearance. The sufferer has 47 chromosomes instead of 46.
Huntingdon's chorea	This involves progressive mental impairment, where the symptoms do not appear until between the ages of 35 and 50.

2. **Are any of these linked to racial groups?**

   Racially linked disorders (both sexes):

Cystic fibrosis	This mainly affects Western Europeans and white Americans. The person is vulnerable to lung

infections and cannot absorb fats and other nutrients from food. Sticky fluid builds up in the nose, throat, airways and stomach and daily physiotherapy is required to clear this. The person is frequently prescribed antibiotics to clear lung infections.

Sickle cell anaemia (See question 1.)

Thalassaemia This is found in people of Mediterranean, Middle Eastern and South East Asian origin. It is a group of blood disorders where there is a fault in the production of haemoglobin.

3. Are any of them linked to the sex of the person?

Sex linked disorders (affecting men only):

Colour blindness Most types of colour blindness only occur in men although occasionally a woman suffers from colour blindness.

Muscular dystrophy This is a slow and progressive degeneration of muscular fibres.

Haemophilia This is a bleeding disorder where a particular blood protein is missing.

4. Do you know of anyone with a terminal illness or who had a terminal Illness? If so, what was it?

(Personal response required.)

5. How would you feel if you knew you wouldn't survive past your 20s, and possibly not even as long as that?

You might feel:

- angry
- as if life had no point
- bitter
- jealous of others
- scared
- that you want to make the most of the time you have got.

6. (a) Are there any genetically linked illnessses in your family?

(Personal response required.)

(b) If so, you may need to go for genetic counselling before starting a family of your own. Why is that?

Genetic counselling is guidance given to a couple considering having children where one or both partners has a blood relative, or previous child, with a genetic disorder. Or the couple might be closely related, such as first cousins, or the woman might be relatively advanced in years for bearing a child or may have had several miscarriages or still births.

7. **If you and your partner were both carrying a serious genetically linked disease, do you think that you would go ahead with starting a family? (With genetically linked diseases, if both partners are carriers, there is a 25 per cent – 1 in 4 – chance of passing the full disease on to their offspring and another 50 per cent – 1 in 2 – chance of making their offspring carriers of the disease. So there is a 25 per cent chance of having a completely healthy baby.)**

(Personal response required.)

8. **If one of your friends had a serious illness, how would you support him or her?**

- Be prepared to spend time listening to the person even if you have heard the same things before.
- Be sympathetic.
- Try to cheer the person up but understand when he or she is moody or wants to be left alone.

9. **Why is it especially hard for parents, guardians and friends to cope with death in a young person?**

- Parents and guardians don't expect to outlive their children. Death is more acceptable in an elderly person who has lived his or her life to the full and may not be in good health in any case. But it seems wrong for a young person, who should have a whole lifetime ahead of him or her, to die.
- Friends don't expect to be faced with death young in life – it might be their first experience of it and would make it harder if they were close to the person.

10. (a) Have you experienced bereavement?

(Personal response required.)

(b) If so, how did you feel?

(See Leader Sheet 5, question 1 for suggestions.)

(c) How would you like to have been supported through your grief?

With patience, acceptance (people grieve in different ways – there is no one 'right' way), sympathy and understanding. (The exercise on bereavement which follows looks at this in more detail.)

Exercise: BEREAVEMENT

Task I

You are friends with Dara, but did not know Heidi. Heidi does die from sickle cell anaemia when she has her next crisis. Cut the following suggestions into strips and put them in order of how best to help Dara cope with her bereavement, with the most suitable suggestion at the top.

1. You avoid Dara as you are clumsy and embarrassed by emotional issues and are worried that you will say the wrong thing to upset her further.

2. Put aside some time to be alone with Dara so that she can talk about her feelings for Heidi and her death.

3. Try to imagine what it would be like for yourself to lose a friend or relation and think of how you would like to be supported if you were in that position – and then support Dara in this way.

4. Tell Dara that she should be glad that Heidi is dead as she is no longer suffering.

5. Ignore Dara's bereavement as much as possible – the less time she has to dwell on Heidi's death, the quicker she'll get over it.

6. Avoid mentioning Heidi to Dara as every time she says something about Heidi, her eyes fill with tears and you can't cope with her emotions.

7. Tell Dara that grief is a selfish emotion as it concentrates on her loss, only unsettles her and does nothing to help Heidi.

8. Tell Dara that you are very sorry about Heidi's death and ask her to tell you how she wants to cope with it, as you will respect her wishes.

9. Remember a year later that Dara might still be suffering from Heidi's death, tell her you haven't forgotten about it and invite her to talk about Heidi and her feelings for her.

10. You believe that Dara should cry a lot to help her deal with Heidi's death, so bring up the subject of Heidi as much as possible.

Task 2

Would your responses to a bereaved friend depend on whether you were dealing with someone of the same sex or someone of the opposite sex? For example, would you give physical comfort to a friend regardless of his or her sex? Explain your answer.

Task 3

(a) How does grief affect a person and how long does it last?

(b) What things help the grieving process?

Task 4

Can you explain how your culture/religion deals with death and grieving? For example, believing that your loved one will be re-incarnated may make death easier to cope with.

Leader Sheet: Exercise on Bereavement

Task 1

Suggested order:

(2)   Put aside some time to be alone with Dara so that she can talk about her feelings for Heidi and her death.

(3)   Try to imagine what it would be like for yourself to lose a friend or relation and think of how you would like to be supported if you were in that position – and then support Dara in this way.

(8)   Tell Dara that you are very sorry about Heidi's death and ask her to she tell you how she wants to cope with it, as you will respect her wishes.

(10) You believe that Dara should cry a lot to help her deal with Heidi's death, so bring up the subject of Heidi as much as possible.

(4)   Tell Dara that she should be glad that Heidi is dead, as she is no longer suffering.

(5)   Ignore Dara's bereavement as much as possible – the less time she has to dwell on Heidi's death, the quicker she'll get over it.

(6)   Avoid mentioning Heidi to Dara, as every time she says something about Heidi, her eyes fill with tears and you can't cope with her emotions.

(9)   Remember a year later that Dara might still be suffering from Heidi's death, tell her you haven't forgotten about it and invite her to talk about Heidi and her feelings for her.

(1)   You avoid Dara as you are clumsy and embarrassed by emotional issues and are worried that you will say the wrong thing to upset her further.

(7)   Tell Dara that grief is a selfish emotion as it concentrates on her loss, only unsettles her and does nothing to help Heidi.

Note:

- Although suggestion 9 is a good one, when someone has died you shouldn't wait a year to show your friend that you care, so it has been placed low down on the list. In reality, there is often much support at the beginning of a bereavement, but later people forget and assume all is going well. Not many would remember a year on that the person might still be hurting, so it is a valuable suggestion.

- Suggestion 4 is aggressive, so is not very high in the suggested order. It would be more appropriate if it were rephrased: You comfort Dara by telling her that Heidi is no longer suffering and has found peace at last.

- Suggestion 6 is low in priority because it concentrates more on the comforter's inability to cope rather than his or her helpfulness to Dara.

- Suggestion 7 is last on the list as it is aggressive and not at all helpful.

Task 2

Would your responses to a bereaved friend depend on whether you were dealing with someone of the same sex or someone of the opposite sex? For example, would you give physical comfort to a friend regardless of his or her sex? Explain your answer.

Responses do vary depending on the sex of the person. If you are a male comforting another male, it is far less likely that hugs and touches are used. Also, men find it harder to cry or show emotion because they have been brought up to be macho and to not display emotions, seeing it as a sign of weakness. Consequently, their relationships tend to be less deep and personal than women's. If a man is going to get emotional and open up it is more likely to be with a woman.

Women are far more likely to give physical comfort to either another woman or a man. They are also more likely to encourage the person to talk about his or her feelings and be prepared to let them cry without feeling embarrassed as their male counterpart might.

Task 3

(a) How does grief affect a person and how long does it last?

A grieving person may become depressed, even suicidal. The worst of the grieving may be over in about two years, but even after that, there can be a great feeling of loss. Even when death is expected, it still comes as a shock. Often there is an initial reaction of numbness or unreality that can last from a few days to several weeks.

Once the period of numbness is over, the bereaved person might constantly think about the dead person; familiar sights, sounds and especially smells reminding him or her. Having conversations with the dead person and laying an extra place at the table by mistake are also common.

After several months, depression might follow where the person loses interest in life, lacks energy, sleeps badly and can experience great weight loss or gain.

Children usually show their grief in a change of behaviour, such as becoming aggressive or angry, bed-wetting or finding it hard to concentrate. It can be hard for some children to express their grief and they may not show any emotion for months or even years.

Chronic grief is a failure to reach the final stage of the normal recovery process – the grief is often more severe and can involve excessive guilt or self-blaming. The person may also feel an overwhelming anger towards the person who has left him or her. Here professional help is needed.

(b) What things help the grieving process?

- Seeing and touching the body of the dead person. (This is very important in helping come to terms with still birth.)
- Attending the funeral helps the acceptance of death. (The grieving person needs to understand that the deceased really is dead and that there is no coming back.)
- Having support on the anniversaries of the death, the deceased's birthdays, Christmas and other important times.
- Seeking help from an organisation such as CRUSE, the National Organisation for the Widowed and their Children. It offers help in emotional and practical matters.

Task 4

Can you explain how your culture/religion deals with death and grieving? For example, believing that your loved one will be reincarnated may make death easier to cope with.

Buddhism	Buddhists believe in reincarnation and that the deceased has been brought one step closer to Nirvana, a state of absolute bliss. Rebirth is influenced by karma – the collective sum of good and evil thoughts, words and deeds in previous lives.
Chinese Taoist	Chinese Taoists believe that after death the soul crosses a bridge to the next life where there are ten courts whose judges decide whether the deceased has had a good life and can pass through the gates into heaven or whether they have to be punished first. Models of worldly goods are burnt during the burial to help souls through the courts.
Christian	Christians believe their deeds in life are judged and, depending on how good or bad they were, they go to heaven or hell.
Hinduism	Hindus believe a person's soul is reborn many times, into other people, or other living things, before it can reach God. The goal of Hinduism is to gain release from this chain of rebirth and merge with the World Soul – Brahmin.
Islam	Muslims believe their soul is looked after by the angel of death in a place called Barzakh until God finally judges the world – then the good go to paradise and the wicked to hell.
Judaism	Jews believe that after their death their soul goes 'to the world that is to come' – the Torah refers to life after death and to a day of reward for the righteous and reckoning for the wicked.
Sikhism	Sikhs do not mourn when someone dies because they believe the dead person moves one step closer to God. They believe that people are born again, but may rest for a while in heaven or hell before coming back to earth.

STORY 37: *Escape!*

Julia checked her watch for the fifth time as she hurried home from the station. Exhausted from her day's work and the over-crowded underground she knew there would only be just enough time to shower and change before going to Dominic's office dinner party.

'You're late,' Dominic accused when she got home. Not, 'You must have had a hard day' or 'Was the train cancelled again?' or 'You must be tired'.

'Yes.' Too tired for a confrontation, she went upstairs to get ready.

'Get that off and put your brown dress on. You're my wife, not a whore.'

Julia was stunned. Dominic had always said how much this dress suited her. She hadn't worn it in their six months of marriage and since no one at his office had seen it, she thought it ideal. It was only slightly low cut. Tears pricked at her eyes. Everyone had seen her old brown dress – he was making her feel like a dowdy old maid with no self-esteem. How could she face all the other wives in new creations while she was wearing such a boring old thing?

'But I thought you liked it?' Julia tried to reason.

'I do. But it doesn't mean everyone else has to see you in it. Now get changed.' He consulted his watch impatiently.

Julia's heart sank. Tonight was going to be an ordeal, smiling and chatting, pretending that they were the perfect married couple. He was always very solicitous when they were in company and made out that all the shortcomings in the relationship were hers.

There had been indications that Dominic lacked trust and was intensely jealous if she so much as looked in the direction of another man – but Julia had mistakenly thought that once he felt more secure with a wedding ring on her finger things would improve. But they didn't. They had got worse.

At work, Julia had a very responsible job where she was well respected and in control of a department. But at home, it was Dominic who controlled her – completely. She had to account for every moment she was out of the house and had had to give up her friends because of him. She used to go out without Dominic but he'd made it so hard for her that it became easier not to go out at all

– he would accuse her of having affairs and would call her names. When she suggested he accompanied her, he refused. It wasn't even possible to invite friends home because he was either openly rude to them or he would tell her that they were leading her astray and were not suitable. Now she was cut off from everyone else and a prisoner in her own home, frightened of incurring her husband's wrath.

'Can I have some money?' Julia asked.

'What for? I gave you some already this week.'

'I spent it on lunches. I didn't fancy sandwiches this week. I need some new shoes.'

'You've got plenty of shoes.'

'But they're old. Two pairs have holes in.'

Dominic grudgingly gave her 25 pounds. Julia knew she'd be lucky to get a new pair for that.

'I do earn it, you know,' she said. They were on equally high salaries.

'Yes, but we agreed that I look after the money so that we save for the future. There won't be your salary coming in when we have children.'

'What do you mean?'

'Well, you'll be giving up work, of course.'

Of course, Julia repeated to herself, that's what he wanted. Then she'd have no excuse to leave the house. She felt the walls of her prison closing in as she visualised the once love-of-her-life holding the key to the prison door aloft, forever out of reach, and she shuddered.

Discussion Sheet 37: Escape!

1. It can take people time to recognise and accept that their partner is controlling them. You may think it will never happen to you or that you will never try to control another person. How do you think you could safeguard yourself against these situations?

2. List all the ways in which Dominic controlled Julia.

3. How did he succeed with these ways?

4. Can you think of any other ways to control a partner?

5. (a) What do you think would happen to Julia if she had children?

   (b) What do you think would happen to the children?

   (c) How would their view of relationships be formed?

6. If your parents or guardians have a similar relationship to Julia and Dominic, or you have a parent or guardian who closely controls you, how has it affected you? Will you fit into the same roles as an adult or try to ensure this does not happen?

7. (a) How did Julia's relationship with her husband affect her personality?

   (b) Were these changes beneficial?

8. Could Julia improve her relationship and make it a more equal and fair one? Give reasons.

9. If Julia decides to escape from the relationship, what should she do?

10. Give examples where you think it would be wise to separate permanently from a partner.

Note: Controlling relationships can be in homosexual, as well as heterosexual, relationships and the controlling partner can be of either sex. Controlling relationships can also exist between parents or guardians and their children.

Leader Sheet 37: Escape!

1. *It can take people time to recognise and accept that their partner is controlling them. You may think it will never happen to you or that you will never try to control another person. How do you think you could safeguard yourself against these situations?*

   You could ensure you are not controlled by:

   - keeping an eye out for controlling behaviour
   - reacting strongly if you think another person is trying to control you just for his or her own ends
   - being careful about moving in with someone – you should know a person well before this happens so that you are not dependent on the person for a home
   - keeping things on an equal footing – sharing out the jobs, money etc. and not giving up control over your own life
   - ensuring you have a get-out if necessary (somewhere to go if things turn nasty).

   You could safeguard yourself from controlling another person by:

   - showing respect towards the other person
   - listening to what he or she has to say and talking over any fears or insecurities you might have
   - treating the other person as an equal with the same rights you expect yourself
   - asking yourself if what you expect is reasonable or whether you have over-high expectations
   - making sure you never threaten or use physical strength to overpower the other person and make him or her give in to your wishes.

2. *List all the ways in which Dominic controlled Julia.*

   Dominic controlled:

   - what Julia wore
   - whom she saw, what friends she could have

- what she did in her free time
- her money.

He also wanted to take control over her having children and make Julia give up work to have and look after them.

3. ***How did he succeed with these ways?***

- He frightened her into submission with his anger. She was frightened he might hurt her.
- He prevented her from having outside contact by accusing her of having an affair and by being rude to her friends, making it not worth her while to go out without him. (But he refused to go with her to see her friends.)
- He made her feel guilty for being late by showing her that he'd noticed and was displeased.
- He controlled what she wore by making her feel cheap for choosing inappropriate clothes, telling her she dressed like a whore and by limiting the money she had to spend on clothes – she had to get his approval before he handed it over.
- He constantly criticised her, lowering her self-esteem, making her less able to fight back or stand up for herself.
- He criticised her in front of others, making out that all the faults in the relationship were hers, demeaning her. Julia would appear foolish if she denied or corrected what he said as it would make her look petty, and she may fear he would embarrass her further. (They were his friends at the dinner party and may barely know her so would not be likely to stick up for her.)
- He didn't allow her to make any social contact with another man, let alone have a platonic relationship with one, as he was intensely jealous. He would punish her for it.
- He controlled her money so that she had to consult him over every expenditure and was not free to go anywhere without his knowledge.
- He made it clear that it was his decision for her to have a baby and give up work. He had no intention of consulting her feelings about it. What he said went. The tone of his voice told her she had no option.

4. Can you think of any other ways to control a partner?

You can also control another person by:

- being moody (if the person doesn't do what you want you can sulk until he or she gives in)
- suggesting he or she is the one with the problem (blaming him or her for everything that goes wrong)
- threatening suicide if the person wants to leave you
- threatening physical harm if the person does not do as you ask
- putting the person down by forgetting important occasions, ignoring or belittling the person, telling the person that he or she is too sensitive or that he or she exaggerates the situation, not taking him or her seriously
- raping the person, forcing the person to take part in sexual acts he or she feels uncomfortable about.

5. (a) What do you think would happen to Julia if she had children?

- Julia said that her husband was getting worse, not better. If she gave up work to have children, she would be completely at his mercy with no regular contact with the outside world and he would probably be even stricter about what she did and whom she saw.
- He might begin to abuse her physically as there would be no one to see her injuries and he would be more confident about his position of superiority. A woman without a job is more vulnerable than a woman earning and independent.

(b) What do you think would happen to the children?

- The children would probably also be tightly controlled and any misdemeanours would be blamed on Julia being a bad mother.
- The children might be psychologically affected, being scared for themselves and their mother, having trouble sleeping and having anxiety symptoms (headaches, stomach aches, nightmares, bed-wetting, inability to concentrate).
- They may be scared to leave their mother at home with their father or be scared of being alone with him themselves.

- They might start to hurt other children, or animals, if they themselves are hurt.

(c) How would their view of relationships be formed?

- They would not have positive role models for relationships and may believe that relationships are not meant to be equal, that it is the norm for one to be very dominant while the other is very submissive. Often people who have had controlling and abusive parents or guardians have controlling and abusive partners themselves.
- They may have difficulty trusting other people and be shy of forming meaningful relationships, fearing getting hurt.
- They may be so used to getting into trouble for the slightest thing that they behave too well, afraid that others will tell them off, and not behave spontaneously.
- They may misbehave out of the home because they are so tightly controlled within it and need to 'let off steam' and work off their frustration.
- When these children have children of their own, they only have their own parents as role models. There is a high chance that they, too, will try to control their own children.

6. *If your parents or guardians have a similar relationship to Julia and Dominic, or if you have a parent or guardian who closely controls you, how has it affected you? Will you fit into the same roles as an adult or try to ensure this does not happen?*

   (Personal responses required.)

7. *(a) How did Julia's relationship with her husband affect her personality?*

   - Julia became more timid and submissive. Although she was earning the same as her husband and had a good job with a high level of responsibility, she was not treated, and was not able to behave at home as, an equal to her husband. Her self-esteem had been dashed and so had her confidence.

- She was not thriving under her husband's care but turning into a nervous and anxious woman with no social network to support her.

(b) Were these changes beneficial?

Not at all. Julia should grow in confidence as she gets older, supported by a loving partner, not become totally controlled by a power-hungry man who is so insecure that he cannot trust his wife at all.

8. **Could Julia improve her relationship and make it a more equal and fair one? Give reasons.**

- Julia could offer an ultimatum – if Dominic did not give her control over her own money and let her live how she wanted, she'd leave him. However, this threat is only realistic if she has supportive parents or friends who could take her in and protect her from her husband should he turn nasty.

- If she has no such support, or if she tried the ultimatum and he threatened her with violence (or physically attacked her), she could seek help from a women's refuge. If he were really nasty, she may have to leave the area and take on a new identity and find new work.

- If Julia were to try to make the relationship equal, she would need to be very careful about starting a family as she might put herself, and her children, at risk. Julia could insist that her husband receives counselling and that they must sit down and talk their problems through. However, Dominic might see it differently and think all the problems are on Julia's side.

9. **If Julia decides to escape from the relationship, what should she do?**

Julia should probably clear out while her husband is at work and go to a safe place where there are people to protect her – or to a women's refuge so that her whereabouts can't be traced. She should probably first seek advice from a women's refuge centre on how to handle the situation.

10. Give examples where you think it would be wise to separate permanently from a partner.

If you:

- are worried about your safety
- are made to do things against your will or that you feel very uncomfortable about
- have no enjoyment from the relationship – the take is all on the other person's side
- are abused (physically, sexually, are not allowed medical attention when you are ill, are punished by not being allowed enough to eat or drink or by being kept cold)
- are not allowed to follow your own interests, career or hobby.

EXERCISE: DECISION-MAKING – ENDING A RELATIONSHIP

If you are not happy in a relationship and are thinking of ending it but are not sure why, or do not think that your reasons will override your need for companionship, set your thoughts down on paper, logically. Do it in private, so that you can be totally honest with yourself to achieve a true answer.

Penny's Dilemma

Penny has been with Dean for nearly two years. He used to be very attentive and affectionate but this has stopped over the last six months. He often irritates her, especially in his over-casual appearance. He is also very untidy, which does not affect her at the moment, but would if they found a place together.

A while back, she saw him punch his younger brother quite hard and the thought that he might be violent has played on her mind, although he has never hit her. Looking to the future, she does not think he would make a good father and knows instinctively that she doesn't want to marry him. (She knows that she definitely would like to be married some day and have children.)

At the moment, that does not present a problem as neither of them has mentioned marriage and Penny knows she does not want to marry in the next few years. She has plenty of time to find someone else. She would quite like to break off from the relationship but knows she will miss him as they do get on very well together most of the time and she does not have anyone else lined up to distract her from a broken relationship. She's worried that she'll end up going back to Dean because of loneliness.

Penny draws up a chart of reasons for staying in the relationship and reasons for going. She knows she will not stay with him for good, but what she does want to know is whether to break it off now or carry on for a while until other factors come into play.

Task 1

How do you view this approach?

Task 2

Look at the chart that Penny has made (on page 316) and assign a score to each point based on the following scale of 1 to 3:

3 = Very important reason

2 = Important reason

1 = Not so important reason

Task 3

1. Does Penny stay in the relationship for now, making an effort to put right what is wrong, or does she have overriding reasons to go?

2. What difference in points is needed to give her a reason to leave the relationship? (A difference of just one or two points is not very significant – it is likely she would go back to him from loneliness or from wanting an escort if there is no great difference.)

Task 4

Dean tells Penny that he has found a place for them to live together. What difference does this make to the scoring? Put the new scores in brackets, next to the old ones affected by this development. What does she do?

PENNY'S RELATIONSHIP CHART

Reasons to stay	Score	Reasons to leave	Score
He's fun to be with.		He's not 'husband' material.	
We get on well – we rarely argue and are never at a loss as to what to talk about.		He's already inattentive. What will he be like after another two years?	
He's reliable.		He irritates me.	
He's sympathetic to my problems.		His show of violence worries me.	
I love him, but not passion-ately.		He drinks a lot and is often drunk.	
He's got a car and takes me wherever I want to go.		He's not ambitious – it doesn't matter that I'm more intelligent, but he's actually lazy and can't be bothered to work or take exercise.	
I've invested two years of my life with him – if I go I'll have to get to know someone else from scratch.		He's from a 'rough' home. Our families would not 'mix'.	
He's the same religion as me so understands a big chunk of me.		I nag but he doesn't take any notice, so I do it more as I get no response. Why won't he listen to me (and stick up for himself)?	
I enjoy the physical side of our relationship.		He wants us to sleep together but I don't want to.	

Leader Sheet: Suggested Scoring for Penny's Relationship Chart

Reasons to stay	Score	Reasons to leave	Score
He's fun to be with.	2	He's not 'husband' material.	2 (3)
We get on well – we rarely argue and are never at a loss as to what to talk about.	3	He's already inattentive. What will he be like after another two years?	2 (3)
He's reliable.	2	He irritates me.	2 (3)
He's sympathetic to my problems.	1	His show of violence worries me.	2 (3)
I love him, but not passion-ately.	1	He drinks a lot and is often drunk.	2 (3)
He's got a car and takes me wherever I want to go.	1	He's not ambitious – it doesn't matter that I'm more intelligent, but he's actually lazy and can't be bothered to work or take exercise.	2 (3)
I've invested two years of my life with him – if I go I'll have to get to know someone else from scratch.	1	He's from a 'rough' home. Our families would not 'mix'.	2 (3)
He's the same religion as me so understands a big chunk of me.	2	I nag but he doesn't take any notice, so I do it more as I get no response. Why won't he listen to me (and stick up for himself)?	1 (2)
I enjoy the physical side of our relationship.	1	He wants us to sleep together but I don't want to.	1 (3)
Totals	14		16 (26)

Leader Sheet: Exercise on Decision-Making – Ending a Relationship

Task 1

How do you view this approach?

It is very sensible to think logically whether it is the best thing or not – it looks objectively at the whole relationship without being swayed by momentary feelings that can swing first one way and then the other. In times of difficulty after the decision has been made, the chart can serve as a reminder as to why you made that choice.

In Penny's case, she wants the best for herself and has not considered that it might be unfair to her boyfriend to carry on going out with him if she knows she definitely doesn't want to marry him. However, it doesn't sound as though he's passionate about her either, so he probably wouldn't be very hurt. And, very often, couples don't break up unless one of the pair finds someone else.

Task 2

Suggested scoring is on the chart sheet.
Notes on the scoring for reasons to stay:

- Penny can have fun and get on well with friends, so Dean's presence isn't vital for that – or for lending a sympathetic ear, although they are all pleasant to have.

- Dean having a car is a matter of convenience to Penny – she wouldn't rate this highly in terms of how she values her relationship with Dean.

- Having to get to know someone from scratch is daunting. But when you're young, like Penny, it is just life. You meet people all the time. This is more of an issue for someone who's been with his or her partner for 20 years, say, where there is much 'history'. Also, she has already said she will definitely leave him at some stage.

- Penny would probably enjoy the physical side of a relationship with other partners just as much. So it's not an overriding reason to stay.

Notes on the scoring for reasons to leave:

- Not being husband material is not important if you're young and you're going out with a partner for fun. No one expects you to marry your early partners.

- None of the scores should be given a three at this stage. Penny evidently doesn't object strongly to his drunken and possibly violent behaviour as she's stuck with him for two years already.

Task 3

1. Does Penny stay in the relationship for now, making an effort to put right what is wrong, or does she have overriding reasons to go?

For now, Penny does stay in the relationship. It's stable in that there are no changes about to be made and she does enjoy his company. She could try and make some minor changes such as asking him to stop doing the things that irritate her or to try to put more 'oomph' into his life. Anything more than this suggests she's serious about the relationship developing further and Penny has made it clear that she definitely doesn't want that.

2. What difference in points is needed to give her a reason to leave the relationship? (A difference of just one or two points is not very significant – it is likely she would go back to him from loneliness or from wanting an escort if there is no great difference.)

Probably a good four points plus makes a significant difference. If there isn't any significant difference, Penny should read through her reasons and check her scoring to see if she has weighted everything according to how she feels. But even then it may not be enough to make her leave.

Task 4

Dean tells Penny that he has found a place for them to live together. What difference does this make to the scoring? Put the

new scores in brackets, next to the old ones affected by this development. What does she do?

Notes on the scoring for reasons to leave once Dean has asked Penny to move in with him:

- It's harder for Penny to meet new people if she's living with Dean and, as she doesn't intend to have a long-term relationship with him, it may not be wise to.

- As Dean is already inattentive, he is likely to take Penny for granted once she moves in with him and so will bother less – and may well be more lazy, expecting her to do the housework and even earn the money to keep him.

- If Penny moves in, she can expect that both families will become more involved because they would visit her and Dean there. This could cause more problems as they don't get on, nor would they approve.

- If Penny's already nagging now, if she moves in with Dean, she is likely to nag more.

- Penny doesn't want to sleep with Dean. This is a big issue if she's to move in with him.

Penny has overriding reasons to leave her boyfriend, when she is asked to find a place with him. It tips the balance and she knows that she must break away from the relationship before it goes further – it is fairer to both.

STORY 38: *Marriage*

Year 11 had just been handed out forms to fill in with regard to their future choices.

'What are you going to do?' Meena asked Cathy and Trudy.

'I'm going to a sixth form college – they're allowed to do what they like in their frees and things. What about you?' Cathy said to Meena.

'I'm doing my 'A' levels here – and if I don't get the grades I want I'll do a vocational course. I haven't decided in what though,' Meena replied.

'I'm getting married, so I don't need to fill this in,' Trudy told them. At times, she felt left out as they were so much better at school than she was. But she'd be doing something they weren't.

'You're mad,' Cathy told her. 'Why do you want to get married at your age?'

Trudy was annoyed. What difference did her age make? 'We love each other.' Cathy and Meena groaned. 'There's no point in waiting any longer because I know Martin's the only bloke for me. We've been going out for two years now,' Trudy proudly reminded them.

'But that's no reason to marry. It just means that no one better's come along.' Cathy sniggered.

'We want to start a family,' Trudy continued, determined there should be something they couldn't scorn.

'Are you pregnant?' Meena whispered, shocked.

'No! But we'll start as soon as we're married.' Trudy felt very important saying this. She would soon be a real adult with a ring, a home of her own, her own child and everyone calling her Mrs Ankley.

Cathy and Meena looked at each other. If they said much more, Trudy would take offence.

'Wouldn't it be sensible to wait until you're older – and have a job first for a while so that you know what it's like to earn and budget?' Meena suggested.

'We can learn as we go along. Together. Anyway, I can't stand living at home any longer – I'm an adult and I want to run my own life. And Martin wants us to marry too.'

'Are you sure you're ready for the responsibility?' Cathy asked. 'My mum had another baby a year ago and I never realised just how much work they give you. She's finding it really hard. I know I couldn't cope with one yet. They cry and cry, even through the night. She never gets a full night's sleep.'

'I'm fit and younger than your mum,' Trudy replied. 'And I'll look after my baby well. I know I can. That's what I want. Are you saying all these things because you're jealous? You haven't ever had a steady boyfriend so you don't know what it's like to want to get married.'

'I don't know either,' said Meena. 'But I know I want to wait as long as I can. I'm not like you, I shan't be able to choose for myself – my parents will choose my husband for me.'

'That's gross,' Trudy told her. 'I wouldn't have my parents tell me who to marry.' Then she remembered she'd only got her mum to tell her what to do – she didn't know where her dad was.

'Even so, my marriage may well last. My parents will find someone good and kind for me. It's the way we do things. Anyway, won't it be terribly difficult having a baby and very little money?' Meena asked.

'My mum did it so I don't see why I can't. People don't wait to get married just because they're a bit hard up.' Trudy felt annoyed with them. Why hadn't they just said congratulations to her and other nice things? Why had they tried to spoil it for her?

Discussion Sheet 38: Marriage

1. Why is Trudy going to get married?

2. Analyse each reason and say whether you think it is sensible. For example, she 'knows' that Martin is the only bloke for her, yet she has a limited view of partners as she has never been out with anyone else.

3. List as many reasons as you can think of why people get married.

4. Divide this list into two: good reasons for marriage and risky reasons for marriage.

5. If you are a heterosexual, under what circumstances do you think you would marry? If you are a homosexual, under what circumstances would you commit to a permanent relationship?

6. If you think you will never marry, or commit yourself to a permanent relationship, what are your reasons for this decision?

7. If a couple have children, do you think it matters whether they are married or not?

8. What do you feel about a lesbian couple having children – where one of them is artificially inseminated, or has heterosexual sex in order to get pregnant? Or two homosexual men adopting a child?

9. List factors that can put strain on a relationship. (Homosexual and heterosexual.)

10. Divide the above list into factors you have some control over and those you have very little or no control over.

Leader Sheet 38: Marriage

---

1. *Why is Trudy going to get married?*

   i)   She felt left out. Her friends were talking about things she couldn't hope to do. She wasn't doing well at school.

   ii)   She wanted to be something her friends could not at that stage.

   iii)   She wanted to be an adult and felt that to be one she had to have a wedding ring, a home of her own, her own child and everyone calling her Mrs Ankley.

   iv)   She couldn't stand living at home any longer.

   v)   She wanted to be an adult in control of her own life.

   vi)   She loves Martin and knows he's the only bloke for her.

2. *Analyse each reason and say whether you think it is sensible. For example, she 'knows' that Martin is the only bloke for her, yet she has a limited view of partners as she has never been out with anyone else.*

   i)   Not sensible. If she wants to feel included, she should try to find something in common with the other girls. If she feels that she's not doing well at school and doesn't want to continue with formal education she could try to get vocational work or a vocational qualification where she can prove her worth. Marriage doesn't do that for you.

   ii)   Not sensible. She should want to be an individual and should not compare herself with her friends. By being herself she will be being something her friends cannot. She needs to build her self-esteem from within herself.

   iii)   Not sensible – all that *will* make her feel like an adult but reality will hit and she may mourn the loss of her youth and the fun she could have had as a single working woman.

   iv)   Not sensible. You don't have to get married any more to escape from home – as was the case a hundred years ago! She could find work and cheap accommodation if that's what she really wanted.

v) Sensible – on the surface. Yet getting married so young can prove to be a mistake – she won't be in control of who she lives with and where she goes and what she spends her money on when there's a tight budget and someone else to consider. And having a baby takes all control out of a young person's life. Her husband can still have his freedom, yet she'll be the one at home without money for childcare to free her for work. She'll find she'd had much more freedom at school with her mum cooking and doing her washing for her, for example.

vi) Not sensible. She can live with him if she wants but she's too young to commit the rest of her life to being with him – and she's had a limited experience of partners. She cannot know that she won't fall in love with someone else later on.

3. *List as many reasons as you can think of why people get married.*
See Question 4.

4. *Divide this list into two: good reasons for marriage and risky reasons for marriage.*
Good reasons:

- You are madly in love.
- You cannot live without your partner.
- You are passionate and enjoy sex within a deeply loving relationship.
- You want to have his or her children.
- You get on extremely well.
- You have much in common.

Risky reasons:

- For convenience.
- To become 'adult'.
- You are or your partner is pregnant.
- It feels glamorous.
- For regular sex only.
- To escape from home.
- No one else has asked or is likely to.

- Your parents or guardians want you married.
- Your parents or guardians want grandchildren.
- You want your own home.
- You want to be looked after or to look after someone.
- Your friends are married.
- You aren't 'good' at anything else.
- You want a mother or father figure.

5. *If you are a heterosexual, under what circumstances do you think you would marry? If you are a homosexual, under what circumstances would you commit to a permanent relationship?*
(Personal response required.)

6. *If you think you will never marry, or commit yourself to a permanent relationship, what are your reasons for this decision?*
(Personal response required.)

7. *If a couple have children, do you think it matters whether they are married or not?*
(Personal response required.)

8. *What do you feel about a lesbian couple having children – where one of them is artificially inseminated, or has heterosexual sex in order to get pregnant? Or two homosexual men adopting a child?*
Reasons why it might work:

- The quality of care should be no different to that of a heterosexual couple.
- Homosexual relationships are just as likely to succeed (or fail) as heterosexual ones.

Reasons why it might not work:

- The child might be teased or bullied at school.
- The child might be embarrassed about his or her parents.
- If the child is not a blood relative of either parent, he or she may feel less close – or the parents may feel less committed.

- The child might feel he or she is not being brought up in a household where he or she can take friends home and be regarded as 'normal'. The child might be ashamed of having parents different to the traditional couple.

- The child may not have a role model of the same sex (but this is true of single parents too).

- Traditionally women are the main carers of children, so it might be hard to accept that two men can take over the role of mother as well as father. There is also prejudice about homosexual men being paedophiles. This is a myth. Some homosexual men are, just as some heterosexual men are paedophiles – but it does not automatically follow that all are.

9. *List factors that can put strain on a relationship. (Homosexual and heterosexual.)*

See Question 10.

10. *Divide the above list into factors you have some control over and those you have very little or no control over.*

Some control:

- If either partner is unable to compromise, the other can patiently point out unreasonableness. This can apply to unequal sharing of household chores and unequal decision-making such as what to spend your money on and where to go on holiday.

- If either partner is insensitive to the other's feelings, he or she needs to learn to listen and understand the other's viewpoint. If there is a lack of communication, where one or both partners cannot share thoughts and feelings, you can go to a marriage counsellor to ask for help with your communication skills.

- If one partner is intensely jealous of, or is controlling of, the other partner it usually shows before marriage so the person could have dealt with it then or not got married. The same might be said for violent behaviour.

- If there is a lack of money both partners could be careful in budgeting and try to get a better job, although this is not always possible. If a partner is out of work, could he or she extend his or her skills through training?

- If one or both partners marry too young and their tastes change or they grow apart, they need to recognise this and be in constant touch with each other so that they 'grow' together.
- If lust is mistaken for love – you need to be sure before you marry why you want to marry. You can have sex without going through a ceremony.
- If one partner doesn't want children – this should be discussed before marriage.
- If your parents or guardians were poor role models, you need to make a conscious effort to change your attitudes and approaches.
- If you have problems with you both getting on with your extended families, you need to talk through these difficulties with your partner without getting too emotional.
- Having too high expectations of marriage – if you were not living in the 'real' world, believing that marriages should be perfect when in fact, they are a compromise. You each need to gain and give a little.

Little or no control:

- Having big differences in education or intelligence, one partner may become bored and impatient, the other miserable from feeling inadequate.
- Having a different religion or a different cultural background or different values to your partner.
- Falling out of love, steadily growing apart.
- Having a challenging child with special needs can be a strain and one partner may have to be a full-time carer.
- Coping with a partner's health problems.
- A partner's job taking him or her away from home for long periods while the other partner is left behind getting lonely.
- If one partner has an affair or if a partner's job presents temptations and opportunities for affairs.
- Having poor living conditions.
- Marrying for wrong reasons – the marriage is not strongly bonded and may not survive problems.

- If one or both of you cannot have children, making you desperately unhappy.
- If you experience still birth or cot death. Such traumas can distance couples.
- Having an unequal relationship. For example, if one partner climbs the social ladder and the other gets left behind, or one partner is bored or ashamed of the other.
- If the wife has a better job than her husband and he cannot cope with the 'role reversal'.
- If you have a workaholic partner or one who has some other time-consuming obsession.

STORY 39: *Trudy's Baby*

Martin Ankley was ready to fall asleep when Trudy told him she was pregnant. She'd said it softly, expecting a cuddle of joy from her husband of six months.

'What?' He sat up and stared at her. He could see it was true. 'Oh, my God.'

Trudy was confused. 'But I thought you wanted a baby.'

'Yes. Sometime.' He thought for a moment. 'You could get it aborted. It's not as though we were trying for one.'

'Weren't we?' Trudy was stunned.

Martin gawped stupidly at her. 'You didn't stop taking the pill?'

Trudy remained silent.

'How do you think we'll manage? I'm on an apprentice's wages, you're working as a sales assistant – and for how much longer?'

'We'll manage. Mum did.'

'I don't want to 'manage', I want to live!'

Trudy visited her mum the next day. Mrs Adams buried her face in her hands. It had all been for nothing. Nothing.

'Aren't you going to congratulate me?'

'Was it an accident?'

'No!' Trudy was indignant. She wasn't stupid, she did know about contraception.

'Why?' Mrs Adams' voice was strangled.

'Because I'm married now, Mum, and that's what married people do. They start families.'

'Not at 17 they don't!'

'You did,' Trudy defended.

'And to what end? So that you'd make the same mistakes as I did?'

'But, Mum, you've done fine.'

'I wanted it to be different for you. I wanted you to have a life of your own. Seventeen years of struggling to bring you up and then you choose, *choose* mind, to have a baby. This is one of the most disappointing days of my life!'

A sob broke from Trudy's mouth. Why couldn't Mum understand? It *would* be different. This baby would have a father.

Seven months into her pregnancy, Trudy gave up her job. Permanent fatigue and raised blood pressure meant she had to be careful. Martin was at home less and less, spending the evenings with his mates in the pub. She used to go with him but she was too tired, especially by the time she'd cooked. Martin should stay at home with her, now that they had to save for the baby, but he said he wasn't giving up on life at his age.

Cathy was busy at college and Meena was on a vocational course in computing and was doing work experience. They didn't have time for her. But she'd show them that what she was doing was just as important, more in fact. She would be responsible for a life.

When Trudy caught Martin staring at her bump, she suggested he felt for kicks or baby's hiccups but he refused every time. He seemed to be really squeamish, although Trudy found it surprising considering the type of jokes he told. She supposed all fathers were at sea where babies were concerned – whereas women had maternal instincts built in. They knew how to look after their children.

Trudy lay in hospital exhausted. She'd spent much of the last two months reading books from the library as Martin hadn't wanted to go to the ante-natal classes put on at the hospital and she wasn't going on her own!

Her mum came and cuddled Alicia before bursting into tears. 'She's beautiful. Absolutely beautiful.' Trudy had known her mum wouldn't be able to resist a baby.

Alicia began to cry. Looking at her watch, Trudy decided she was ready for her next feed. She'd been told to change the nappy before the feed so that Alicia could fall asleep immediately after being fed without being disturbed. But eight times a day? By the time her baby was changed and fed and then settled down, it was almost time for the next feed. And babies didn't know the difference between night and day.

Trudy watched as her adorable baby sucked and made little snorting noises. Just like a baby pig! She'd decided to bottle-feed so that Martin could share the work. And Martin wouldn't like having her boobs shown in public. Besides, she'd always wanted to hold a bottle – her doll had had one when she was a child.

After feeding, Trudy placed Alicia back in the tilted cot (because she kept possetting) and hoped Martin would bring more clean clothes as Alicia was wearing her last Babygro.

Having been home for a week, Trudy admitted to herself that it was hard looking after a baby.

'Is your husband helping at all, Trudy?' the midwife asked. Their studio flat was a tip. There was only the one room, apart from the kitchenette and the bathroom.

'He's busy working,' Trudy defended, not wanting to admit the truth.

'It's his child too. Who does the cooking?' Trudy paused for too long so the midwife guessed the truth. 'You must eat, Trudy. I'll ask the health visitor to call, to see what help she can give.'

Trudy didn't want any help. She just wanted to be left alone. She was so unimaginably tired she didn't feel like eating. She couldn't sleep because as soon as she dropped off the baby would cry and she couldn't keep up with the washing. Martin wouldn't take the clothes to the launderette so she had to wash them out by hand, but they still smelt of sick and poo. And they took ages to dry as there were no radiators, only a heater that ran on a meter. And they hadn't the money for that.

'Martin, you must stop spending money on beer. We need it for the baby.'

'It's your baby. I wasn't asked if I wanted one. You sort out the money. Ask for more benefit.'

But Trudy didn't want to do that. They might take the baby away from her, they might say she couldn't look after Alicia properly. Besides, she wasn't entitled to more money.

She looked down at her breasts. If it wasn't for the vouchers, she'd be spending many pounds a week on baby milk – for a whole year!

When her mother called round, she was shocked at how badly her daughter was managing. 'Go and shower while I tidy up.' The sight of Trudy, barely 18, but looking as haggard as a sick woman in her 40s who'd not washed for a week, filled her with complete dread over her daughter's future.

The kitchenette was piled high with grimy unwashed mugs, plates and cutlery. The floor was sticky, the walls were splashed. There were no clean towels or tea towels. The baby's bottles were floating in murky water in the washing-up bowl. Smelly nappies overflowed the bin. Trudy's mum placed her hand over her mouth and nose and quickly opened the window.

The main room was littered with clothes. Trudy's nightwear had become her daywear and stank. Mrs Adams found a black bin liner and filled it with the offending garments. She cleaned, tidied, washed up, sterilised bottles, made up more feeds, changed Alicia, fed her, put her down to sleep and took the clothes to the launderette to be washed and dried while she shopped.

By the time she got back, it was late afternoon and Alicia was being fed again. Mrs Adams placed the folded washing in a pile on the table. Then she cooked a stew.

'You should have called me,' her mum said. 'Told me you couldn't cope.'

'You managed without help.'

'That's because I had to. No one does it by choice. Why isn't Martin doing more?'

'Oh, Mum,' Trudy wailed, 'I don't know what to make of him. I thought everything would be all right once the baby had been born. He stays away for as long as he can.' And he never touches me, she thought. 'I don't think I can carry on.' Her voice wavered before tears flowed.

Trudy cried for an hour, while her mum held her, saddened. Where had she gone wrong? She wouldn't have wished this on her daughter at any price.

Once the torrent was over Trudy's mum promised to help at weekends, when she wasn't at work. 'Until you're back on your feet. Martin will feel better about the baby when he sees how well you're coping.' At least, Mrs Adams hoped so.

But it wasn't until the baby was six months old that Martin took an interest in his child. Trudy had always attended to Alicia's needs. Martin hadn't got up once in the night to help. But tonight was different. 'Martin?' He was immediately awake, recognising the note of panic in her voice. 'There's something wrong with Alicia. You've got to call the doctor, now!' Alicia sounded like a rasping seal and was crying hoarsely in between the racking coughs as Trudy held her fiery body close, calming her. Quickly, Martin pulled on his trousers and a jumper, searched for change and the doctor's number and ran out to the call box.

He came running back. 'The doctor's on her way,' he panted. 'I'll heat up some water in a pan and put the kettle on. We've got to steam her.' Panic stricken, Trudy sat with the crying and coughing Alicia on her knee while the room became misty with steam.

'Let me hold her.'

'You'll drop her.'

'I won't. Please.' He wanted to hold her, he needed her. This tiny, defenceless baby, whom he'd rejected. She was a part of him and he was her dad. Silently, Trudy handed Alicia over, wondering why it took near death for Martin to acknowledge he had a daughter. By the time the doctor arrived, the worst was over. Alicia was still distressed but her seal-like barks had subsided.

'It's croup,' the doctor informed them after a quick examination, giving them a powder to mix with sterile water and a prescription for the morning. 'It's just a precaution, in case she develops an infection on her chest. It won't cure the croup, so you have to be prepared for this to happen again. Steam her like you did this evening or wrap her up and take her out into the cold night air. But if there's no improvement, or if she turns blue, call an ambulance. Hospital staff can give her medication to inhale to reduce the inflammation of her airways. Unfortunately, a baby who's had croup can have recurrent attacks every time she gets a cold – they grow out of it when they're older, when their larynx is bigger.'

Trudy nodded in understanding. She'd been so frightened, she couldn't imagine having to go through it again. And again. How would she have coped with a child that had special needs?

Their marriage had no miraculous revival but Martin developed a resigned acceptance to their way of life, although never showing the same warmth towards her as when they were first married. She'd made a mistake but would be the last to admit it to her husband or her mum. But she did not regret Alicia.

Trudy only wished Alicia had come five years or so later. When she'd worked out her own life first. She'd owed it to herself – a shame she hadn't realised it at the time. She, herself, was important, not merely having status through her role as mother or wife as she'd supposed. That's what her mum had wanted, she understood that now. Looking down at her baby, Trudy fervently hoped that Alicia would recognise her own value and importance as an independent being. She would work towards that and pray she didn't fail – as her mum had with her.

Discussion Sheet 39: Trudy's Baby

1. Why was Trudy's mum upset about her daughter's pregnancy?

2. Trudy had expected her mum to be pleased about her pregnancy – just as she had her husband. Why was this?

3. Does it make a difference that Trudy's baby would have a father, as Trudy claimed?

4. Was Martin really squeamish about Trudy's pregnancy?

5. Is it true that women naturally have built-in maternal instincts and know how to look after their babies?

6. What problems did Trudy have in her pregnancy? Which of these had she brought on herself?

7. What do you think about Trudy's decision to bottle-feed Alicia?

8. What is it like to care for a new-born baby?

9. Why did Martin suddenly become interested in his daughter?

10. What have you learnt from this story?

Leader Sheet 39: Trudy's Baby

1. *Why was Trudy's mum upset about her daughter's pregnancy?*

- Because she had been pregnant at 17 and knew what hardships there were and the sacrifices she had had to make. She didn't want Trudy to have to go through the same thing.

- She wanted her daughter to have a life of her own before she was tied down with babies. She'd gone straight from school to getting married and now was pregnant but had not yet done anything with her life.

2. *Trudy had expected her mum to be pleased about her pregnancy – just as she had her husband. Why was this?*

There must be a lack of communication between Trudy and her mum and Trudy and her husband. If she had had long involved chats with her mum, she would have known how her mum felt about teenage pregnancy and what it was really like. And to get pregnant without first discussing it with her partner was rather silly. Martin had a right to know what she was up to – and in becoming pregnant, she had also irrevocably changed his life too, without his permission.

3. *Does it make a difference that Trudy's baby would have a father, as Trudy claimed?*

It would if the father were a willing dad, and if he's likely to stick around for a long time. Although Trudy and Martin have been together for some time, it is well-known that teenage relationships are less likely to last and become a long marriage because personalities, outlooks on life and expectations can change so much during the more youthful years. Trudy would have been better off waiting until they both decided that they wanted to start a family. It also puts less strain on a relationship if the couple earn enough money to have some spare after necessities and for emergencies, and to live in a warm and comfortable place.

(Although Martin was earning, he was on a low wage. Had Trudy been on her own, she would probably have received more benefit making either circumstance equally financially challenging.)

4. *Was Martin really squeamish about Trudy's pregnancy?*

No – Trudy told us he wasn't squeamish because of the jokes he told, although she preferred to believe he was, as the alternative was unpalatable. Martin didn't want to have anything to do with Trudy's pregnancy and would have liked to deny the existence of a developing baby. By distancing himself from Trudy and her tummy at this time, he showed he didn't want to be part of what was going on.

5. *Is it true that women naturally have built-in maternal instincts and know how to look after their babies?*

There is some truth in it but not to the extent that Trudy believed. Mothers find it hard to leave their babies to cry – the cry of a baby is designed to make a mother pick up her baby to cuddle and see to his or her needs. However, most of mothering has to be learnt, hence ante-natal classes, advice given by midwives, health visitors and doctors, and the numerous books and magazines on the subject.

However, not all mothers naturally take to their babies. There may be some problem such as post-natal depression where the mother is at risk of neglecting or even harming her baby. Trudy has a simplistic view on life and, because she didn't look into the idea of mothering beforehand, really does not know what to expect.

Note: Trudy felt that men were 'at sea' when it came to looking after babies. This is a sexist viewpoint. Men are as capable of looking after babies and children as women (although they have the biological drawback of not being able to breast-feed). It is stereotyped attitudes and lack of expectation that puts men forward as incapable child-rearers. Trudy was happy to perpetuate this myth because she wanted something that she could do better than anyone else – hence her reasons for leaving education and getting married in the first place (as mentioned in *Story 38: Marriage*).

6. *What problems did Trudy have in her pregnancy? Which of these had she brought on herself?*

Problems brought on by herself:

- Martin's non-acceptance of becoming a father.
- Martin's resentment of her.

- Not having sufficient money – they were both on a low income before she was pregnant so she knew they were on a tight budget.
- Being left on her own while Martin carried on with his life like a single man with no responsibilities. It was a natural reaction for him to have given that he hadn't wanted the baby and the resultant pregnancy wasn't through his carelessness.
- Her mother's disappointment in her. If she'd talked her intentions over with her mother, she would have realised how her mother had felt.
- She was lonely because her friends were busy getting on with their lives and she was stuck at home, too ill to work and too tired to go out with Martin.

Other problems:

- Her high blood pressure.
- Having to stop work before she'd expected to.

7. What do you think about Trudy's decision to bottle-feed Alicia?

It was made for the wrong reasons. She should have been thinking of what was best for her baby, not whether Martin ought to be sharing the work. This is another thing she hadn't discussed with him and it's not something she can change her mind about later. If she doesn't breast-feed in the first few days, her breast-milk will dry up. It doesn't seem she took much in during her reading on mothering, and she could have gone alone to the ante-natal classes. Midwives are very pro breast-feeding so that babies can acquire immunity to illnesses from their mothers and Trudy could have picked up on this from either source.

Trudy also had a sweet childish view of babies – that they lie quietly in their mother's arms while they drink. But they also squawk, are sick, and do not care if you need a sleep or that it's the middle of the night. Trudy thought feeding her baby would be like feeding a doll.

8. What is it like to care for a new-born baby?

Hard work and very tiring. If the baby is premature, he or she may need feeding every two hours (twelve feeds a day). If the baby is born when expected, he or she will need to be fed every three hours. You also have to change the baby's nappy before feeding – eight changes a day, and feeding can take up to forty-five minutes. You then have to wind the baby after feeding, or the baby will be sick and have tummy ache when you put him or her back to bed. So, in between feeds, you have far less time than three hours, having only the chance of snatching sleep throughout a 24-hour period. In between these times your baby can cry because of tummy ache (and may be sick, requiring a complete clothes change), boredom, not feeling as secure as being in your womb or because he or she is hot or cold or tired. And in between all this you need to eat, sleep, wash yourself, wash your baby's clothes and yours and so on. This goes on for the first six weeks or so without a break.

9. **Why did Martin suddenly become interested in his daughter?**

- Because he was at risk of losing her. He felt guilty that he hadn't taken an interest in her or held her, and feared that now it might be too late.

- He had been punishing Trudy by not becoming involved with Alicia but finally realised he'd also been punishing himself by denying himself the right to be a father and denying Alicia too – the poor defenceless baby who hadn't asked to be born.

10. **What have you learnt from this story?**

- The importance of communicating with the people around you.

- That the decision to have a baby should be taken by both people concerned after thought and discussion.

- Not to rush into things.

- To research what you intend doing thoroughly – this will give you a greater chance of a positive outcome.

- To enjoy life and make yourself secure before you deliberately take steps to make yourself vulnerable. And then make sure you have support where possible – it's extremely hard to 'go it alone' like Trudy's mum had done.

- That having a baby is not as simple as it can appear. Many problems can occur during pregnancy, in childbirth itself and after childbirth, with both mother and baby. Either or both might not be well, or the baby might not be as perfect as hoped.

- To understand that having a baby can affect the relationship you have with your partner, regardless of whether he or she agreed to starting a family.

- The folly of believing that babies are like dolls and that you are playing 'houses' when you marry. It's far more serious and the consequences more long-term than that.

- What a huge responsibility it is to bring up a child, and that the decision should never be taken lightly – the child's, and your, happiness is at stake.

STORY 40: *The Last Straw*

Patrick sat in McDonald's nibbling French fries. He had the entire day to himself as he did every Saturday. Earlier, his mum had asked, 'Have you done your homework?' He was 18 and resented being treated like a child. That he was certainly not – he'd got through the death of his father, hadn't he? Put up with his mum's emotionless stony silences, denying shared grief?

'Nearly. I'll finish tomorrow.' He'd worked hard all last night and now only had an essay to write. His mum had nodded, satisfied, opened her mouth and quickly closed it again, checking herself.

What had she wanted to ask or say? Patrick wondered abstractedly. Was he meeting a friend? She should know the answer by now, for he had no friends. It was a difficult thing to admit to but it was true, despite moving to college, hoping for a fresh start. It seemed it wasn't bad luck that had made his school friends ridicule him, describe him as effeminate, accuse him of being gay, tease him mercilessly about his studious nature, his desire to succeed. It was him.

Girls had giggled if he'd talked to them, even to ask them for their essays when he collected them for the teacher. No one had taken him seriously or befriended him. His only use had been to lend his homework for the scrutiny of others too lazy or busy to do their own. Until he'd stopped it. He wasn't a doormat. But they'd been more derisive, fuelling their judgement of his homosexuality, laughing at his heated denials, taking pleasure in harassing him.

Patrick had been brought up in a devout Christian family but the very God his parents had taught him to worship had denied him the all-important gift – that of making friends. It was the only thing he cared about.

Loneliness stalked him day and night, peaking on weekends when he lacked the company of his peers, bustling happily around him, seldom interacting with him. The students had quickly decided on their friends, formed cliques and needed no more, leaving Patrick on the outside looking enviously in. Would it be like this for him all his life? A friendless, sterile life? He had no reason to think otherwise.

Gradually, Patrick noticed that there were two girls, of about his age, sitting at the corner table, only a few feet away. One was crying, the other had her arm comfortingly around her friend's shoulder, her face showing sympathetic concern.

Patrick had no fear of being caught gawping as he had long since learnt that he was invisible. People looked through him as though he didn't exist, was of no consequence. It was as though he were seated outside, looking in through a one-way window.

Many a time he'd wanted to shout, 'Look at me! I'm a person! I've got feelings too!' Instead, his frustration was corked inside, requiring a detonator to unleash the pent-up anguish he felt. One day his deepest emotions would become unstoppered and he looked forward to having the ability to express himself, but feared the effect it would have. For then, he could not justify his continued existence as his dislike of the world and his raw despair would be for all to see.

He clenched his fist, willing himself not to think like that, for people would think him mad if they only knew what wretched thoughts he harboured. And that may well be worse than being considered gay – which he was not. He got an erection as often as any bloke his age did faced by an attractive girl, judging by the conversations he'd heard.

Patrick watched as the girl's tears were dried and saw her smile shyly at her friend. If only his own hurt could be assuaged so easily. Boys were not permitted the luxury of crying in public – it was simply not done. And who would dry his tears?

Suddenly, he knew what he had to do to break the circle of misery – he'd thought about one particular way out for more than two years and at that moment the appeal of killing himself was too great to ignore. And he knew why – he had no vestige of pride left and strangely, this gave him the courage he needed, before his chance was gone.

The girls had shown him that everyone needed someone and as he had no one, there was but one thing he could do to save himself. His mum had told him his life was just beginning, that he had everything to live for. But he knew he had nothing. Nothing at all.

He knew where to go. He'd passed it often enough. Leaving the girls and French fries behind, he walked a while, stopped, took a deep breath and took the most important step of his life. He entered the building of the befrienders of the desperate, the Samaritans.

Discussion Sheet 40: The Last Straw

1. (a) Why did Patrick go to the Samaritans?

   (b) What else could Patrick have done to improve his situation?

2. (a) Suggest reasons why male suicides are far more numerous than female suicides.

   (b) What could be done to reduce male suicides?

3. (a) Why do people ridicule, humiliate or act in a hostile manner towards others for no 'real' reason?

   (b) Is it right to gain pleasure at the expense of others?

4. (a) How do you think an ostracised (left-out) person feels?

   (b) Have you, at any time in your life, experienced this in some way? If so, how did it make you feel and what, if anything, did you do about it?

5. (a) How would you feel if you knew you had contributed to making someone feel desperate enough to take his or her own life?

   (b) If you have been behaving unkindly and unfairly to someone, what could you do to put things right?

6. (a) Could you tell if your behaviour (or someone else's) towards a person was having a dangerous effect?

   (b) Should you be wholly responsible for your actions (and inactions)?

7. Were you disappointed that Patrick went to the Samaritans instead of killing himself? Why?

8. (a) How does our culture or upbringing, or the effects of television and other media, teach us how to behave?

   (b) Why don't we, as a nation, act more kindly to others?

9. (a) Respect, empathy, sincerity, trustworthiness, being non-judgemental and a good listener are some of the qualities a counsellor needs. What do they involve?

   (b) Do you have any of these? (If not, would it be a good idea to try to develop some?)

10. (a) Who would you go to if you were in trouble? (Who would you not go to?) Would you seek guidance from an outsider? Who would be affected by your suicide?

    (b) Is it right not to give people a chance to put things right? (They may have no idea you're unhappy.)

Leader Sheet 40: The Last Straw

1. **(a) Why did Patrick go to the Samaritans?**

   - He was desperate and had no pride left to prevent him from going.

   - He was ready to admit to someone else that he needed help, and that he was friendless and lonely.

   - He was depressed and could see no light ahead of him, feeling pessimistic about his future.

   - He was afraid he was going to harm himself.

   (b) What else could Patrick have done to improve his situation?

   - He could have gone to his mother, sat her down and made her listen to how he felt. He could have asked her to be more open with him and their relationship may have reached a new understanding, the event bringing them closer together instead of driving them apart as the death of his father had.

   - If Patrick were religious, he could have gone to his religious leader for support.

   - He could have sought counselling from an organisation that helps the bereaved come to terms with their loss.

   - He could have gone to see his doctor. Patrick was obviously depressed and doctors know that this poses a suicide risk. As well as listening to Patrick, his doctor may have prescribed anti-depressants and referred him to a psychologist, to help him through the difficult time.

2. **(a) Suggest reasons why male suicides are far more numerous than female suicides.**

   - Boys and men can feel under pressure to be 'macho' and life can be made hard for them if they don't behave according to stereotype. Some consider it manly to bully, deriving fun from sexist, racist or anti-gay jokes. The romantic and caring side of boys' personalities is usually suppressed to conform to well-established role models rather than risk being ridiculed themselves, putting pressure on those boys who cannot, or find it hard to, conform to society's expectations. This makes them feel threatened and failures as 'men'.

- Boys and men are not usually brought up to express their feelings and to show emotion publicly, so often have to bottle it up to show a brave face to the world whereas society is tolerant of women and girls being emotional and sharing their problems.

- Boys and men do not tend to talk over emotional issues or discuss relationships with their fathers, who might expect them to 'fight their own battles'.

- Male friendships tend to differ from female friendships in that they are less intimate. Boys and men don't tend to discuss the details of the ups and downs of their lives and do not generally expect to get emotional support from a fellow male. This is particularly true if their father is absent or will not discuss emotional problems, whereas female friendships tend to be more caring and supportive, and involve the sharing of deep fears and worries. They also tend to involve more physical contact than male-to-male friendships.

- Suicide is a form of violence – against the self. Many boys and men who are suicidal have had experience of violence at home or in school (or both) and may become violent themselves when they are in distress, seeing this as a way to deal with problems. They are also more likely to have been in trouble with the police.

- Young men are also more likely to deal with stress by using alcohol, drugs or cigarettes to relieve it and, while under the influence of these, may feel less inhibition about acting violently against themselves. Young women and girls are more likely to react to stress through having anxiety disorders such as an eating disorder, although in recent years there has been a marked increase in teenage girls drinking and smoking.

- Suicidal young men are more likely to keep their problems to themselves and withdraw, staying in their room. They are at greater risk if they do not live in a supportive family structure, such as living in care or a hostel or being homeless.

- If the young men are lonely and do not have friends or supportive friends, they are at far greater risk if their mother is absent, as she can be a great support.

- Suicide is a greater risk if the person has low self-esteem. Many young men might feel threatened by the equality of women and feel uncomfortable having to compete with the opposite sex. They feel, as men, that they should be the strongest (emotionally and physically) and the more intelligent – otherwise their 'manhood' is threatened.

Far more young women than young men attempt suicide, but their attempts tend not to be as desperate and therefore not as successful as men's.

(b) What could be done to reduce male suicides?

Male suicides could be reduced by:

- Encouraging boys and men to discuss emotional issues with their male friends and offer intimacy and understanding that are assumed to be qualities of women.

- Improving boys' and men's listening skills by teaching them to listen without interruption or feeling they have to dominate a conversation. (It's not a competition.)

- Challenging sexist or other stereotypical remarks made by others and ensuring you don't use them yourself.

- Helping to increase boys' and men's self-esteem by showing you value and respect them when they do something praiseworthy.

- Showing boys and men that emotional support is better than using alcohol, drugs or cigarettes to solve their problems or relieve their stress.

3. (a) Why do people ridicule, humiliate or act in a hostile manner towards others for no 'real' reason?

Doing this is a form of bullying. The person behaves in this way to make him or herself feel big and powerful – yet it is actually cowardly to take advantage of someone who is unable to stand up for him or herself. Such people think only of themselves. They are immature in that they do not recognise that they must take responsibility for the things that they do and say.

(b) Is it right to gain pleasure at the expense of others?

No, although you may feel this is justified as a form of revenge if the person has wronged you in some way – but in this story, Patrick has wronged no one. Sometimes a person will tease someone they are fond of as a natural part of a close relationship but it has nothing to do with the pleasure being one-sided, leaving the other person deeply hurt and offended.

4. **(a) How do you think an ostracised (left-out) person feels?**

Being ostracised is extremely lonely and greatly affects your self-esteem. You might feel worthless, of no consequence, invisible (as Patrick did), unloved, uncherished, bitter and angry with the world. You might feel that life holds nothing to interest you and that it is pointless to go on. You might get very depressed and not care about eating properly or dressing yourself smartly or keeping yourself clean. No one can thrive in an environment where there are no rewarding experiences. The importance of friendships in someone's life cannot be over-valued.

(b) Have you, at any time in your life, experienced this in some way? If so, how did it make you feel and what, if anything, did you do about it?

(Personal responses required.)

5. **(a) How would you feel if you knew you had contributed to making someone feel desperate enough to take his or her own life?**

You might feel:

- guilty
- responsible
- shocked
- horrified because you had no idea the person felt like that
- desperate to make amends.

(If you felt happy about the fact that you contributed towards someone's wanting to kill him or herself, you would be very mean. Not too many would want you for their friend.)

(b) If you have been behaving unkindly and unfairly to someone, what could you do to put things right?

- You could tell the person you had not intended him or her to feel so bad and that you feel terrible about it. To you it had only been a bit of fun and you hadn't realised the effect it would have.

- You could apologise and say that you will never behave like that again and could you be friends? (You don't have to be best friends, but you could certainly 'look out' for the person in the future and stop to chat whenever you see him or her.)
- You could ask about the person's feelings and what else had made him or her feel this way.

6. **(a) Could you tell if your (or someone else's) behaviour towards a person was having a dangerous effect?**

Probably only if you observe the person and notice changes in his or her behaviour. For example, he or she might:

- become moodier or more aggressive
- become unresponsive to taunts
- purposely isolate him or herself from others
- give up any pretence of trying to take part in social interactions
- take less care of him or herself
- behave differently such as being overly cheerful
- appear very tired
- eat more or less than usual
- talk about there being no point in going on.

(b) Should you be wholly responsible for your actions (and inactions)?

If you have deliberately set out to make someone miserable, for no good reason, when that person is obviously in a vulnerable position, like not having friends to counteract what you do and say, then yes – you should be wholly responsible for what you do and fail to do. You are no longer a young child who knows no better. You are an adult and with that comes responsibility for your own behaviour.

7. **Were you disappointed that Patrick went to the Samaritans instead of killing himself? Why?**

Yes: Because it was an anti-climax. The story made you think that he was going to kill himself, so it was a rather 'soft' ending.

No: It would be tragic that so young a life was extinguished just because it was going badly for him at that time. His father had died and he was obviously still suffering – he should have had counselling long before now to help him cope with it. The Samaritans are specially trained and used to dealing with desperate people. It's what they're there for and Patrick had nothing to lose by giving them a chance to help. How would his mother have coped, losing her son as well as her husband? And she would always blame herself for her son's death, for not noticing how miserable he was inside because she was too caught up with her own grief.

8. **(a) How does our culture or upbringing, or the effects of television and other media, teach us how to behave?**

- Our culture is shaped by our religion, using its values to show us how to behave. For example, Christians are supposed to be caring towards others, forgiving and generous with their kind deeds.

- Some people are brought up to think themselves superior to others and so may not look favourably on any but a chosen few. Other people have been brought up by an abusive adult who shows little care. This might make the person want to bully and be aggressive towards others. Our home environment contributes to the way in which we behave, but it depends on how susceptible we are to it – members of the same family can be very different. Not all can be blamed on home life. Once we become adults we should make our own decisions and take the consequences. It is possible for some positive changes to be made, although many people may need help.

- The effects of the media can desensitise us to what real people feel. We see much suffering around the world on the news, but because we've seen it all before, we are less shocked or concerned by it. Films can portray tough men who please themselves and think to hell with everyone else. They can portray women like this, too, but not to the same extent. We are also often prejudiced. For example, people may believe that those suffering from a mental illness are dangerous, remembering snippets from the media, without understanding that there are different types of mental illness.

(b) Why don't we, as a nation, act more kindly to others?

- Our family structure is different to what it was years ago – more often we live away from parents and grandparents who have less input in the lives of their children and grandchildren.

- Neighbourliness has been reduced. It is more the case that we live without getting to know our neighbours or go round to help when something's wrong.

- We are living in a multi-ethnic society. Many of us do not bother to get to know and understand people from other ethnic groups to ourselves. This creates a barrier between groups of people, who consequently have nothing to do with one another.

- We are more concerned with looking after ourselves than worrying about the well-being of others.

- We tend to live further away from the workplace so do not closely socialise with our colleagues. Years back, people did not 'commute' like they do today, so everyone in a community knew one another.

- Religion is becoming more dilute. Far fewer people go to church and the religion of ethnic groups outside their country of origin is at greater risk – second-generation children do not as closely associate themselves with that culture or religion.

9. (a) Respect, empathy, sincerity, trustworthiness, being non-judgemental and a good listener are some of the qualities a counsellor needs. What do they involve?

Respect

This involves listening to what someone has to say, not putting him or her down, and treating the person as an equal. It involves accepting the person's feelings and thoughts without trying to change them.

Empathy

This involves mentally and emotionally putting yourself into another person's position, trying to understand what it feels like to be him or her with these problems.

Sincerity

This involves meaning what you say, being genuine.

Trustworthiness

This involves keeping confidences and not using the information you are given for your own ends.

Being non-judgemental

This involves accepting the person for what he or she is, and accepting the person's actions without criticism or ridicule.

Being a good listener

This involves being able to listen without interruption and being comfortable with silences should they arise so that the person is free to carry on speaking after having time to think. It is also important to repeat back to the person the situation described so that your understanding is confirmed, and to look interested, giving your whole attention to the other person.

(b) Do you have any of these? (If not, would it be a good idea to try to develop some?)

(Personal responses required.)

10. (a) Who would you go to if you were in trouble? (Who would you not go to?) Would you seek guidance from an outsider? Who would be affected by your suicide?

(Personal responses required.)

(b) Is it right not to give people a chance to put things right? (They may have no idea you're unhappy.)

Ideally you should give people a chance to put things right. The effect a suicide has on family and friends is huge and everlasting. (And the risk of suicide with other members of the family consequently increases.) Suicidal bereavement is intensified by guilt and shame, thinking that others must blame them for what has happened. Also, they get less support from others because people don't know what to say to them and so avoid them. This makes them more isolated and again makes it worse for them. People seem to be more able to offer sympathy and support if the death is from natural causes rather than at the person's own hand.

Religion may also make suicide harder to deal with. For many, it is considered sinful to take one's own life. The family left behind may have this additional burden to bear.

Appendix: Useful Contacts

The contacts listed here are to give help, support or information relating to areas touched on in the book. Many of the organisations listed have local offices. Look in your phone book or ask the head office to give you details of the relevant organisation closest to you. Be prepared to hear a recorded message when ringing out of hours and be prepared to have to keep trying to get through. Many of these lines are very busy and not all will be manned all the time. If you are contacting the organisation by post, include a stamped addressed envelope.

Although address and telephone details apply only to readers in the UK, the listed websites can be accessed from all over the world.

AIDS and HIV

National AIDS Helpline
Tel: 0800 567 123 (24-hour)
Website: www.aidsmap.com

Positively Women
347–349 City Road
London EC1V 1LR
Tel: 020 7713 0444
Helpline: 020 7713 0222
Website: www.positivelywomen.org.uk

(Provides free and confidential practical and emotional support to women with HIV and AIDS.)

The Terrence Higgins Trust
52 Gray's Inn Road
London WC1X 8LT
Tel: 020 7831 0330
Helpline: 020 7242 1010
Website: www.tht.org.uk

(Promotes understanding of HIV and AIDS. Publishes a wide range of free booklets.)

Alcohol Abuse

Alcohol Concern
Waterbridge House
32–36 Loman Street
London SE1 0EE
Tel: 020 7928 7377
Website: www.alcoholconcern.org.uk

(Produces a wide range of publications and online there are links to other useful sites.)

Alcoholics Anonymous
General Service Office UK
PO Box 1
Stonebow House
Stonebow
York YO1 7NJ
Tel: 01904 644026
Website: www.alcoholics-anonymous.org.uk

(Has online information and local contact details, supporting anyone trying to overcome a serious drinking habit.)

Drinkline
Petersham House
57A Hatton Garden
London EC1N 8HP
Tel: 0800 917 8282

(Offers information and self-help materials and support to drinkers, their families and their friends.)

The Portman Group
7–10 Chandos Street
Cavendish Square
London W1G 9DQ
Tel: 020 7907 3700
Website: www.portmangroup.co.uk

(Established by leading drink companies to promote sensible drinking, reduce alcohol-related harm and develop a better understanding of alcohol misuse. Publishes a wide range of material.)

Bereavement

Cruse Bereavement Care
Cruse House
126 Sheen Road
Richmond
Surrey TW9 1UR
Tel: 0870 167 1677

Website: www.crusebereavementcare.org.uk

(Offers help and counselling to the bereaved.)

Bullying

Advisory Centre for Education

22 Highbury Grove
London N5 2DQ
Tel: 020 7354 8321

(Publishes information sheets on bullying and runs a helpline.)

Anti Bullying Campaign

185 Tower Bridge Road
London SE1 2UF
Tel: 020 7378 1446/7/8/9

Bullying Online

Website: www.bullying.co.uk

Kidscape

2 Grosvenor Gardens
London SW1W 0DH
Tel: 020 7730 3300
Website: www.kidscape.org.uk/kidscape

(Aims to keep children from harm or abuse before they become victims.)

Parentline

Highgate Studios
Highgate Road
London NW5 1TL
Tel: 020 7284 5500
Helpline: 0808 800 2222

(Helpline for parents about many issues, including bullying.)

Child Abuse

American Academy of Child and Adolescent Psychiatry

Website: www.aacap.org/publications/factsfam/index.htm

(Publishes online fact-sheets on issues affecting children.)

ChildLine
2nd Floor, Royal Mail Building
Studd Street
London N1 0QW
Tel: 020 7239 1000
Helpline: 0800 1111 (24-hour)
Website: www.childline.org.uk

(Publishes online fact-sheets on issues affecting children.)

ECPAT UK (End Child Prostitution, Child Pornography And the Trafficking of children for sexual purposes)
Website: www.ecpat.org.uk

(Campaigns for British legislation to be amended so that it protects all children, both in the UK and overseas, from commercial sexual abuse.)

International Child Abuse Network
Website: www.yesican.org/definitions.html

(Information on child abuse.)

Kidscape
(see Bullying)

NSPCC (National Society for the Prevention of Cruelty to Children)
National Centre
42 Curtain Road
London EC2A 3NH
Tel: 020 7825 2500
Child Protection Helpline: 0808 800 500
Website: www.nspcc.org.uk

Counselling

British Association of Counselling
1 Regent Place
Rugby
Warwickshire CV21 2PJ
Tel: 01788 578328

(List of counsellors all over UK, information and advice.)

The Samaritans
10 The Grove
Slough
Berks SL1 1QP
Tel: 01753 216500

National helpline: 08457 909090 (24-hour)
Email: jo@samaritans.org
Website: www.samaritans.co.uk

(Gives help to people who feel suicidal or desperate for any reason.)

Youth Access

1–2 Taylors Yard
67 Alderbrook Road
London SW12 8AD
Tel: 020 8772 9900

(Gives local contact details of services for children and adolescents, including counselling and advice, information and befriending.)

Drug Abuse

ADFAM National

1st Floor Chapel House
18 Hatton Place
London EC1N 8ND
Tel: 020 7405 3923

(National charity for families and friends of drug users.)

Drug and Alcohol Concern

Colindale Avenue
London NW9 5HG
Tel: 020 8200 9525

National Drugs Helpline

Tel: 0800 77 66 00
Website: www. nationaldrugshelpline.co.uk

(Gives free and confidential advice.)

Eating Disorders

Eating Disorders Association

1st Floor Wensum House
103 Prince of Wales Road
Norwich NR1 1DW
Tel: 01603 621414
Helpline: 01603 765050
Website: www.edauk.com

(Information and support for sufferers of anorexia, bulimia and other eating disorders and their families.)

Ethnic Minorities

Commission for Racial Equality
Elliot House
10–12 Allington Street
London SW1E 5EH
Tel: 020 7828 7022
Website: www.cre.gov.uk

(The CRE works with individuals and other organisations against prejudice, discrimination and racism.)

Institute of Race Relations
2–6 Leeke Street
Kings Cross Road
London WC1X 9HS
Tel: 020 7837 0041/2010
Website: www.irr.org.uk

(This organisation conducts research and produces educational resources to bring about racial justice in the UK and overseas.)

Legal

Crisis Counselling for Alleged Shoplifters
PO Box 1982
London NW4 4NX
Tel: 020 8202 5787

(Helps anyone, including children, accused of shoplifting with legal or medical advice or counselling.)

Citizen's Advice Bureau
Look in your local telephone directory for details. You can get all kinds of legal advice, free of charge.
Website: www.adviceguide.org.uk/nacab/plsql/nacab.homepage

Mental Health

MIND
National Association for Mental Health
Granta House
15–19 Broadway
London E15 4BQ
Tel: 020 8519 2122
Information Line: 020 8522 1728 or 08457 660 163
Website: www.mind.org.uk

(Information service, books and pamphlets on many aspects of mental health.)

National Phobics Society
Zion Community Resource Centre
339 Stretford Road
Hulme
Manchester M15 4ZY
Tel: 0870 7700 456
Website: www.phobics-society.org.uk

(Information and support for phobias, anxiety, panic attacks, compulsive disorders.)

SANELINE
199–205 Old Marylebone Road
London NW1 5PQ
Tel: 0345 678 000
Website: www.comcarenet.co.uk/sthches/saneline.htm

(Helping people cope with mental illness.)

Pregnancy and Contraception

Abortion Help World Directory
Website: www.abortion-help.com

British Pregnancy Advisory Service
Guildhall Buildings
Navigation Street
Birmingham B2 4BT
Tel: 0121 643 1461
Tel: 08457 304030 for details of your nearest branch.
Website: www.bpas.org

(Pregnancy testing, emergency contraception, counselling, help with unwanted pregnancies, abortion.)

Brook Advisory Centres
Studio 421
Highgate Studios
51–57 Highgate Road
London NW5 1TL
Helpline: 0800 0185 023
Website: www.Brook.org.uk

(Help and advice on contraception, pregnancy testing and sexual problems.)

Family Planning Association
2–12 Pentonville Road
London N1 9FP
Tel: 020 7837 5432
Helpline: 020 7837 4044

Website: www.fpa.org.uk

(Provides a nationwide information service on contraception and reproductive health including service provision.)

Marie Stopes International
153–157 Cleveland Street
London W1P 6QW
Tel: 020 7574 7400
Helpline: 0845 300 8090
Website: www.mariestopes.org.uk/msi_worldwide.html

(Provides pregnancy testing, counselling and abortion services and contraception.)

National Abortion Campaign
The Print House
18 Ashwin Street
London E8 3DL
Tel: 020 7923 4976
Website: www.gn.apc.org/nac

(Defends women's reproductive rights and the rights of women to make their own decisions.)

NHS Direct
Tel: 0845 4647 (24-hour)
Website: www.NHSdirect.nhs.uk/main.jhtml

(Health information and advice.)

Sexual Health

The Toxic Shock Syndrome Information Service
24–28 Bloomsbury Way
London WC1A 2PX
Tel: 020 7617 8040 (24-hour pre-recorded information about the illness.)

Sexuality

Albany Trust
280 Balham High Road
London SW17 7AL
Tel: 020 8767 1827

(Personal counselling service for people who are unsure of their sexual identity. Fees are negotiable.)

London Lesbian and Gay Switchboard
PO Box 7324
London N1
Tel: 020 7837 7342
Website: www.llgs.org.uk

(24-hour helpline for lesbians and gays.)

Smoking

ASH (Action on Smoking and Health)
102 Clifton Street
London EC2A 4HW
Tel: 020 7739 5902
Website: www.ash.org

(Provides information on all aspects of tobacco and campaigns to reduce the unnecessary addiction, disease and premature death caused by smoking.)

NHS National Smoking Helpline
Tel: 0800 169 0 169

QUIT (The Stop Smoking Charity)
Victory House
170 Tottenham Court Road
London W1T 7NR
Tel: 020 7388 5775
Quitline: 0800 00 22 00

(Helps people give up smoking and has educational resources.)

Solvent Abuse

Re-Solv (the Society for the Prevention of Solvent and Volatile Substance Abuse)
30A High Street
Stone
Staffordshire ST15 8AW
Tel: 01785 817885
Helpline: 0808 800 2345
Website: www.re-solv.org

(Publishes booklets and videos about solvent abuse and can let you know of local agencies that can help.)

Victim's Support

The Roofie Foundation
Monkswell House
Manse Lane
Knaresborough
North Yorkshire HG5 8NQ
Tel: 0800 783 2980 (24-hour helpline)
Website: www.roofie.org.uk

(This is a voluntary organisation awaiting charity status to raise awareness of the dangers of drug rape and to help and counsel victims. Date rape drugs have the street name 'roofies'.)

The Suzy Lamplugh Trust
14 East Sheen Avenue
London SW14 8AS
Tel: 020 8876 0305
Website: www.suzylamplugh.org

Victim Support
Cranmer House
39 Brixton Road
London SW9 6DZ
Tel: 020 7735 9166
Supportline: 0845 3030 900
Website: www.victimsupport.org

(Counsels victims of crime.)

Women's Support

London Rape Crisis Centre
PO Box 69
London WC1X 9NJ
Tel: 020 7837 1600
Website: www.rapecrisis.org.za

(Counsels victims of rape and sexual violence.)

Women's Aid Federation
9 Orchid Street
Bristol BS1 5EG
Tel: 0117 977 1888
Helpline: 0345 023468

(Offers counselling, practical help and a refuge for women and children who are suffering any kind of harassment, abuse or violence.)

Index of Subject Areas

The subject indicated may be brought up in the story itself or in the questions or answers following that story.

* Titles are connected with other stories. See the introduction to the relevant section to find out the order in which these stories should be read. (The questions in these stories can refer back to previous happenings as there is an underlying theme in addition to the problems that relate directly to that particular story.)